PRAISE FOR JULIE GLYNN

"It's a very rare woman indeed whose life has not been 'tainted' by any insistent mean girl living in her mind. This mean girl tells her that she mustn't enjoy life and isn't worthy of joy, comfort, love, or freedom until she's a size 8, or 4, or 0— or until …. fill in the blank. The list is endless. The only way out—to the meaningful and joyful life you were meant to live—is to recognize that mean girl and outwit her. And that is just what Julie Glynn's book does so masterfully. Read it and show your inner mean girl the exit ramp. You'll be so glad that you did."

— CHRISTIANE NORTHRUP, M.D., NEW YORK
TIMES BEST-SELLING AUTHOR
OF *GODDESSES NEVER AGE, THE WISDOM
OF MENOPAUSE,* AND *WOMEN'S BODIES,
WOMEN'S WISDOM*

"In a culture where we are conditioned to be *so mean to ourselves*, Julie's book is important reading. It reminds us that our inner Mean Girl is trying to keep us in the vicious diet cycle. This book shows you how to break out of that cycle and learn to eat without guilt or regret."

— CAROLINE DOONER, AUTHOR OF *THE
F*CK IT DIET*

"Julie Glynn's book offers a refreshing message to women who are ready to make peace with their bodies. Her practical, fun activities provide a path to living with more freedom and joy, and who doesn't want that?"

"With a simple replicable tool, Julie teaches us how to listen and then convert the 'nasty mean girl voice' we all have in our heads. She shows us how to live fuller and no longer hold ourselves back for (previously unchecked) fear or shame or doubt. This book teaches a simple tool that can quite literally change how you think about yourself and relate to the world."

"I absolutely loved this book. It was Insightful, supportive, real, and touching. I loved the mix of fictional and nonfictional stories. Your two arrows in the shape of a bottom is so smart. I feel this encapsulates the book in a caring and welcoming way as well as the well-known question 'does my bum look big in this.' A delightful read, so real and beautifully written."

— CINDY SHAMES, BUSINESS RESULTS
COACH

"Take a journey and learn to 'befriend Mean Girl.' Julie integrates concepts from Health Coaching and Cognitive Behavioral Therapy to help you find your 'silver lining' and take control of your mean girl."

— BARBARA L. BONNEY, MSN PMH APRN

"To say this book was a fun and emotional ride is, to say the least. You won't regret picking it up, trust me. I'm hoping you'll read it once and keep going back to it whenever you need that extra support and reassurance because Julie will give you the tools to grow stronger from the inside out, and to become a more genuine version of yourself. Julie will teach you how to relate to your thoughts and feelings in a different way, so you can use your actions to move towards the kind of person you want to be and to the kind of life you want to live. Go prepare some hot chocolate and get ready for your next adventure!"

— MARIANA MOLL

IF MY ASS WERE SMALLER LIFE WOULD BE PERFECT

And Other Lies The Mean Girl in Your Head Tells You

JULIE GLYNN

Believe in yourself
and enjoy the journey~
you're worth it ♡
Julie Glynn

Cover design: Andrea Schmidt

Back cover photo: Cara Dyke

ISBN: 978-1-7361168-1-4 (ebook)

ISBN: 978-1-7361168-0-7 (paperback)

Contact Julie: JulieGlynn@yahoo.com

JulieGlynn.com

For my family.

Where would I be without your undying love, support and brutal honesty?

Probably wondering around aimlessly.

Everything I do, I do for you with love in my heart for all of you.

CONTENTS

Introduction   xi

CHAPTER 1   1
Mean Girl Lie:
Everything Is Totally Hopeless

CHAPTER 2   13
Mean Girl Lie:
I can't do anything right

CHAPTER 3   23
Mean Girl Lie:
My thoughts are out of control

CHAPTER 4   35
Mean Girl Lie:
I'll always be a victim of Mean Girl

CHAPTER 5   41
Mean Girl Lie:
I'm Fat and Nobody Likes Me

CHAPTER 6   51
Mean Girl Lie:
I'll Never Measure Up

CHAPTER 7   65
Mean Girl Lie:
I'm not as good as everyone else

CHAPTER 8   75
Mean Girl Lie:
If everyone else got their shit together I could be happy

CHAPTER 9   89
Mean Girl Lie:
If My Ass Were Smaller, Life Would Be Perfect

CHAPTER 10   107
Mean Girl Lie:
I'm not smart enough. I'll fail

CHAPTER 11   121
Mean Girl Lie:
I don't have enough motivation or willpower

CHAPTER 12   135
Mean Girl Lie:
I can't be trusted around food

CHAPTER 13   153
Mean Girl Lie:
I'm Always Going to Be a Failure

Want More?   167
Join Me in Creating Social Change   169
Acknowledgements   171

INTRODUCTION

When I have a choice to make, it helps if I identity what I don't want. For example, when we rebuilt our house—more on that later—eliminating what I did not want made it so much easier to choose the perfect features for me. That being said, I'm going to start by telling you what this book is not. This is not a diet book. I don't support diets. I'm putting this right up front because I want it to be the first thing you see. You will not learn any tips or tricks on how to flatten your tummy or reduce the amount of food you eat. You will, however, be presented with strategies and techniques to learn how to accept the tummy you have and the rest of your body for that matter, regardless of its size, shape, or appearance. You'll also find information about Intuitive Eating, which includes learning how to eat without restriction.

This book is not intended to deal with traumatic experiences or related issues such as PTSD. Additionally, this book is not meant to treat eating disorders. If you are experiencing intense feelings or trauma, you have an eating disorder, or you have significant dieting or food issues, seek appropriate professional assistance. This book does not substitute for the advice of a doctor or other health care provider. However, if you are working to improve your life by changing your thought patterns, keep reading.

This is a book for women who are done dieting or who are ready to give it up but haven't taken the plunge yet. This book may not resonate with you. You may not agree with my views about dieting. That's not to say if you're still dieting you won't find some useful information within the pages of this book. You will.

I started this book by telling you what it's not. When I was field testing titles, I got feedback suggesting I avoid pessimistic language. "Avoid using words like *not* or *don't*; they have negative connotations." However, sometimes positive, encouraging words like *self-love* and *self-care* just don't describe what we really need. Sometimes things seem more clear when we figure out what we don't want and go from there. Perhaps you want to stop being so damn mean to yourself. Or you want to stop feeling guilty about what you eat. Or you want to stop looking in the mirror and feeling discouraged. Or you want to stop hearing that voice in your head tell you that you're a bad person. That's what this is about.

This book is based on the idea that we all have that voice in our head that sabotages us. I call the voice *Mean Girl*. "If your ass were smaller, life would be perfect," is an example of a lie Mean Girl might tell you. You know what I'm talking about?

That voice in your head that repeatedly shames and minimizes you with comments like:

"You'll never amount to anything."
"You shouldn't be eating that."
"That wouldn't have happened if you made better choices."
"You'll never measure up."

I've personified the voice in your head as Mean Girl to help you better relate to it, accept it, and neutralize it. When Mean Girl is left to her own devices, she is not a trustworthy guide for you. She will try to keep you stuck in the same old cycles and keep you from growing and developing as a person. However, she can be turned around, and we're going to work on that throughout this book.

One of the ways we're going to do that is to look at a new cycle you can apply that will help you not only address Mean Girl, but also help you gain control of the thoughts that create the emotions that lead to your actions that create your results. I call this process the Silver Lining Cycle because it helps you gain both clarity and control so you can create thoughts that best serve you in any situation.

MEET DARLENE

Darlene is going to take this journey with you. She is a fictional character who has a variety of experiences to share: some positive, some negative, some heartbreaking, and some revolutionary. Her stories and details are a compilation of actions and situations either from my life, my friends' lives, or my clients' lives. I created her to help illustrate common feelings many women share. Darlene is here to remind you that you are not alone. Darlene is a tough cookie, but she doesn't believe that. She lacks confidence, but with just the slightest shift, she could be quite the firecracker. She's a learner, grower, nurturer, and she's open to change and experimentation. Darlene has a kind, gentle heart, and she's loving and caring. She's willing to be in touch with her feelings and needs. She struggles with her weight and self-image, and she's been on every diet there is.

Darlene is looking for something to help her feel more worthy—to increase her happiness and self-acceptance. She knows the answers are out there; she just doesn't know where to find them. She's willing to take the reins and do what she needs to do; if only she knew what that is.

As you read through Darlene's experiences, you may find things that resonate with you and things that don't. Please take what you like and leave the rest. Not everything that worked for Darlene is expected to work for everyone.

NOW MEET JULIE

Today I stand in front of you as a confident, self-loving, body-accepting woman. There are probably more than just a few people reading this book shaking their head saying, "Wow, things sure have changed."

Things weren't always and aren't always smooth sailing. I'm not perfect. Throughout the book, I will share some of my struggles and the strategies that worked for me. You can apply them in your own life and see how they can work for you.

So how did I get where I am now? I have two master's degrees. The first one is in special education, which allowed me to work with a wide range of students who taught me more about thinking, emotions, behaviors, and consequences than any degree program could have. My second master's is in health and wellness coaching, which taught me how to help guide others in finding and navigating their path to self-discovery in order to live their life to its fullest. I've been a member of Self Coaching Scholars for two years, and I'm also a Certified Intuitive Eating Counselor and a Be Body Positive Facilitator. I don't share any of this to brag, but to help illustrate the components that, combined with my life experience, helped me neutralize my mean girl and come to terms with my own body.

Finally, let's talk about my writing style and the layout of this book. You're probably thinking, "With two degrees she's probably a real stickler for grammar and punctuation." Um, no! I'm a conversationalist, and I like to write as if I'm talking to you. Because of that, I might start some sentences with "or," "and," or "but." I might even end some sentences with a preposition. I don't know. It doesn't matter. The point is this method works. But enough about me.

There are a lot of activities and strategies sprinkled throughout this book. I know, you're groaning like a student who just found out there's a pop quiz. I confess, I don't always do the suggested activities presented in books, mostly because I never want to stop and get a sheet of paper. I like to binge read. You can do that if you want, but if you do, I encourage you to go back and do the activities later. It's part of this system I created, and it's beneficial for you to not only do them but also to keep them in a journal or a folder where you can go back and reference them later. So go grab some paper and let's get started. *Or, if you are holding the printed book, use the Notes section at the back of the book.*

❧ I ❧

MEAN GIRL LIE:

EVERYTHING IS TOTALLY HOPELESS

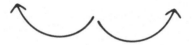

The first draft of this book wasn't at all like what you're currently holding in your hands. It contained a lot of fluff and filler and just a tiny bit of substance. I emailed that draft to my content editor friend, and a few weeks later, I traveled out of town to attend her wedding. After the wedding, we hugged and promised we'd finish working on the book when she returned from her honeymoon. Things didn't turn out quite the way we had anticipated. The very next day my life turned upside down, and I became a completely different person.

That experience brought an entirely new perspective to the message of this book. I share my story more openly with you in this version, not so you'll feel sorry for me but to demonstrate that the ideas in this book can work whether life is smooth sailing or a complete wreck.

The day my life flipped over started on Long Island at my sister-in-law's house. About ten minutes after we left her house to start our journey home, she called and said we forgot our pillows (actually, my pillows; my husband doesn't really care about bedding). If we went back, we'd be late meeting my other sister-in-law for breakfast. I didn't want to be late, so I seriously thought about leaving the pillows and just buying new ones when we got home. I'm so glad we decided to go back for the pillows.

Around noon that same beautiful July day as we continued heading home, we were on the ferry boat between Long Island and Connecticut. I rested my head on my husband's leg while I lay on a bench on the deck and enjoyed the bright light and warmth of the sun mixed with a cool breeze. I remember thinking everything was perfect. I was startled when my phone rang, but I ignored it. Soon after, a loud horn sounded, followed by a muffled voice requesting passengers return to their cars as we prepared to dock in Connecticut. My phone beeped indicating the caller left a message. Curiosity prompted me to listen to the message as I navigated the noisy crowd back to the car. Holy shit. It was the police.

Our house was on fire!

They calmly informed me, "The room downstairs, where you first enter, is really bad. The rest of the house, upstairs, is just smoke damaged."

Whew! Just smoke damaged. That was great news, especially since our living space, kitchen, and bedrooms were all upstairs. We'd clean that up in no time.

I asked, "Can we sleep there tonight?" The officer paused, and in a sad and compassionate tone, he said, "No. I'm sorry. You won't be able to sleep there." He added, "We've contacted the Red Cross on your behalf, and they will be in touch with you soon."

I didn't say it, but thought, "We don't need to get the Red Cross involved. We can stay at my daughter's for the few days it takes to wipe down the smoke."

Soon after I hung up, a friend called from our front yard. I asked him to text me pictures of the house.

He said, "No."

What? People don't usually tell me no. I pushed then he admitted, "Seeing pictures will just make you more upset."

The four-hour ride home felt like four days. I cried my eyes out between countless phone calls. I remember in one quiet moment, I noticed this excruciating pain from my throat all the way to my pelvic bone. I just wanted to open my mouth and scream. I knew that wouldn't make the pain go away, plus it would probably scare the shit out of my husband. Tears were gushing and I pleaded, "I don't want this to be real. I don't like the facts; they hurt, and I want to change them."

When we finally arrived home, we found cars, fire trucks, and people lining our street and an overpowering smell of smoke. Our house, our yard, and the cars in our driveway were cordoned off with police tape; even we weren't allowed to cross. I learned it was called in around 11:30 a.m. and fire departments from three different towns responded. It was after 7:00 p.m. when the last fire truck finally left.

A young firefighter sitting on the back of one of the trucks told me, "When we pull up to a fire in the middle of a weekday and see two cars in the driveway and there aren't any homeowners standing in the yard, we go inside and look for bodies."

What a horrible thought. But how fortunate, not only were we not home, but our little doggie was at daycare, and she had her bed with her. Whew, we had pillows, and she had a bed.

I remember lying awake in a hotel room most of that first night feeling lost, confused, and homeless as tears rolled from my eyes down the side of my head and into my ears.

The next day we were allowed to go inside. I learned a whole new meaning of the phrase "just smoke damaged." I can't begin to describe the devastation the smoke left behind. I felt violated as I walked through our home and saw how invasive smoke is. The entire inside was ruined. Damn smoke. The house needed to be gutted down to the studs then rebuilt. So much for just wiping things down.

In the weeks that followed the fire, I cried. I cried a lot. I could have cried more. Sometimes I wish I had cried more.

Sometimes I felt like I couldn't possibly cry more. My chest hurt. It was tight. I was uncomfortable. I felt hungry and I felt full at the same time. I was tired, yet I couldn't sleep. I experienced the physical effects of emotional pain. I noticed it. I felt it. I didn't like it. I acknowledged it. I wanted it to go away. I looked around, unsuccessfully, for some way to control these feelings. Some way to change this situation that hurt so much.

Fire isn't something that happens one day and then you pick up the pieces and start moving on the next. It takes days and weeks and months of sifting through ash, burned rubble, and documenting and replacing your loss while trying to acclimate and create a home in temporary housing, sleeping in a bed that's not yours (at least I had my pillows). You find yourself looking for things you don't have and mourning again and again for things you didn't realize you lost. I didn't know how long I could stand it. I needed something. I wanted something, anything, that would help get me through it.

A week after our fire, I was stopped at a red light. When the light turned green, I had to wait while three blaring fire trucks came through the intersection. As I sat in my car, I started to cry. Just one week ago at almost the exact same time, these fire trucks were racing to my house.

That's when I noticed it. Right in the midst of this horrible moment when I was so desperate for some kind of relief. It came after practicing many of the strategies I share in this book, and it was the first time I really noticed the significant change in Mean Girl's voice in my head. At first, she was silent. Then I heard something different than what I was used to hearing. It was kind, warm, and loving. She spoke softly and asked, quite simply, "Who do you want to be right now? Do you want to be a victim, or do you want to be a survivor? It's totally up to you. This can be an opportunity for you to grow if you want to."

I chose survivor.

I didn't know exactly how to do that, but based on my skills and expertise, I knew it started with my thoughts. As a matter of fact, when I cried out in the car on the way home that I didn't like the facts and I wanted to change them, I knew then that my thoughts could change everything, but I was not in a place to do anything other than experience my feelings.

A couple of weeks after our fire, I went back and reviewed an old Facebook post a coach friend had posted. He called it "10 Reasons My Flight Delay was the Best Gift Ever." I decided I would try it. Of course, it was far too outrageous calling our fire "the best gift ever." I settled on just calling it a gift. Making this list was one of the hardest things I've ever done. I struggled. I cried. I thought deep and I thought hard. I'm sharing this list with you as an example of how to look deep for the silver lining of an unpleasant situation.

TEN REASONS WHY THE FIRE WAS A GIFT

1. I experienced, firsthand, the kindness and

compassion of others. It helped me learn the value of receiving. I'm more aware of the importance of providing care and compassion when someone else experiences hardship.

2. I identified and endured feelings of emotional pain in my body. I sat with it. I didn't try to buffer or escape those feelings. In a short amount of time, much less than I expected, the feelings weakened until they eventually went away. I know now that I can handle/manage emotional pain, and I don't need to be fearful of experiencing it in the future.

3. I have the level of strength I always hoped to have. I had the wherewithal, in a time of crisis, to recognize I had a choice to make, and I made the best choice for me. I found my strength, and I became the person I want to be. I chose not to feel sorry for myself and not to get lost in letting others feel sorry for me either. I chose to face forward and made sure that every single day, we were moving in the right direction.

4. I believe there is a silver lining in everything. No matter how horrible something appears, it could be worse. I get to choose how I want to view every situation I face. Whatever it is I choose, is exactly what I'm going to see.

5. I have a renewed gratitude for the health and safety of my family and pet. It's easy to take the wellbeing of our loved ones for granted. However, it's something we need to cherish on a daily basis.

6. No one was at fault. Two investigations concluded

the fire was an accident. I accepted that. I didn't blame anyone. I didn't blame myself. My entire life, I've always thought I was responsible for every bad thing that ever happened to me. Not this time. Not anymore. When there's no fault and no blame, there's no guilt or regret.

7. We were remodeling at the time of our fire. We made a few mistakes, common in most do-it-yourself projects. There were a lot more things we wanted to do. Many things we probably never would have done. That's all changed. Putting our house back together will be like an HGTV fixer-upper show where they demo the entire inside of the house and rebuild it. When the house is done, there shouldn't be anything I'll want to change, fix, or paint.

8. Some emotional blocks about what I feel I "deserve" have been challenged. I didn't think I deserved people caring about me. I didn't feel like I deserved a nicely finished house. I believe this disaster happened for a reason, and one of those reasons was a hard slap on the head that I do deserve the level of care and compassion I've been shown. I do deserve all the blessings I've received.

9. I experienced the joy of showing my appreciation for the people who helped. All the workers who had a hand at cleaning and rebuilding our house were a gift. It was a pleasure trying to brighten their days through silly conversations and stories, treats, or surprise lunches.

10. All the clutter is gone. Things that needed to be

discarded or donated are no longer taking up space. I don't have any closets, boxes, or bins that need to be sorted out. This frees up my time to spend on more enjoyable and productive things.

It's important to mention, I didn't just make this list, then my life was all fine and dandy. I still get angry and grieve and feel overwhelmed and exhausted. Just the other day, I went looking for something I don't have anymore, and all those feelings came back. The list was a useful standby to help shift my thinking when I get stuck too long holding on to feelings that don't serve me.

NOW ABOUT MEAN GIRL

Don't get me wrong, Mean Girl still comes around, and she can be snarly, but she's much more subtle, and her jabs are less debilitating than they used to be. For the most part, she's loving and supportive. She teases me when I do silly things rather than belittle me.

She wasn't always this way. She was as mean as any other Mean Girl. I can't blame her. I believed everything she said without question. I believed her when she said I was to blame for every discomfort I experienced. I even believed her when she'd make ridiculous claims like, "You got a bad grade on that exam because you're fat." It wasn't a physical fitness test; it was an entrance exam. But I believed her because I believed that women who fit the media's mold for beauty never experience pain. They are happy and smart. They have effortlessly clean houses, great jobs, children that don't talk back, marriages without arguments, large savings accounts, and tons of friends, and I have never been one of those women who fit that mold. I've since discovered all the diets, dye jobs, nail salons, and workouts in the world will never make you so thin and pretty that you're free from heartache and discomfort.

One thing I know with 100 percent certainty, this fire had absolutely nothing to do with the size of my ass. In fact, nothing that ever went wrong in my life had anything to do with my size or weight. As a result, the topic of weight is now off-limits with Mean Girl. She is no longer allowed to blame anything on my size or weight ever again.

All these years, we've let Mean Girl create misery. Maybe it's time we turn her around and let her create some happiness and security for us instead. Imagine having a constant ally who reassures you and cheers you on, asking questions like, "Who do you want to be? How can I help?" Calming you with statements like "Don't worry, you've got this."

It can happen without experiencing a house fire. You, too, can become friends with Mean Girl. It just takes time and practice. I'll help you.

* * *

ACTIVITY:

To start with, next time you experience something that creates uncomfortable feelings, take out a sheet of paper, and see if you can come up with a list of reasons the situation is a gift. You don't have to come up with ten reasons. If you do, great, if not, don't worry. Take a minute and look at my list again. You can use some of my ideas as a springboard for your list: gratitude, silver linings, blame, compassion, and appreciation.

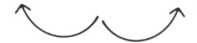

✣ 2 ✣

MEAN GIRL LIE:

I CAN'T DO ANYTHING RIGHT

I've never really liked the saying, "Well if it's meant to be..." It feels like an excuse to sit back, do nothing, and just wait and see what, if anything, happens. I've always been more of a "make it happen" kind of gal. The "wait and see" method conflicts with my personality.

Then I came across this idea—what if it was "supposed to happen?" At first, it sounded a little too much like "If it was meant to be." But the more I thought about it, the more I realized it felt kind of liberating. If things were supposed to happen, then they weren't my fault. I could stop feeling guilty, stop torturing myself, and stop wasting energy beating myself up, and finally accept the fact that I can't change the past. I can, however, change the way I think about it, how often I think about it, and how much of it I bring into my present and future life. I can also decide whether to use my previous experiences to my advantage or as an excuse. We have no way of knowing how things would have turned out if they hadn't happened the way they did. All we know for sure is that they happened. Maybe they were supposed to.

Sometimes people ask if I regret not being home at the time of our fire. Maybe it wouldn't have been as bad if we'd been home, suggesting maybe we would have been able to put the fire out ourselves before it caused so much damage. I dunno. Then I think, what if we were home and asleep? What if we didn't get out? What if we got out but couldn't save our dog? What if we were home and had to run out with just the clothes we were wearing? I wouldn't have had my purse, phone, license, credit cards, shoes, or clothes; all the silver linings I happened to have with me on the long weekend away. What I do know is that it happened exactly the way it was supposed to happen.

You might be thinking, "That's easy for you to say. You were lucky. Things turned out okay for you. Some of us have gone through really serious shit, and there's just no way we could possibly believe it was supposed to happen the way that it did." I know. I get it. Throughout this book, I am going to ask you to look deep inside in order to grow. I share some of my most serious experiences as an example and an inspiration to show that it can be done.

Enduring a house fire was pretty traumatic. But it's not the most traumatic experience in my life. My most traumatic experience happened when I was just nineteen years old.

It was late afternoon on a sunny Tuesday in May. I was immediately confused when I pulled in to our huge, Y-shaped driveway after work and saw my dad and brother awkwardly leaning against the back of the car in our opened garage. My brother didn't live at home, so that was strange. Even more peculiar was seeing my aunt looking out our kitchen window. She lived more than thirty minutes away and never visited on weeknights.

I knew right away something was wrong. I just didn't know what. I couldn't even guess. All I knew was I wanted to avoid it, whatever it was. I got out of my car and stood there. I started questioning my dad for an explanation of these oddities. He asked me to come over closer. He said he wanted to talk to me. No! I wasn't going any closer. I hoped if I kept a safe distance between us, he couldn't tell me anything bad. I wanted this thing, whatever it was, to go away. Right now! I even thought about getting back in my car and driving away. Then there wouldn't be anything wrong. My anxiety was high and justifiably so.

My mother died that morning.

It's really hard to wrap your head around death, never mind trying to see it as something that was "supposed to happen." It's an even more incomprehensible, impossible, maddening idea when death is a suicide.

Mean Girl stood up front and center. "This is your fault," she declared. "You caused this. You should have done something to stop it."

She went on to accuse me, "You're mouthy and arrogant. Your room is a pigsty, and you eat too much junk food."

Mean Girl told me all the reasons it was my fault. "You argue. You don't listen. You never apply yourself. You'll never amount to anything."

On and on she went:

"You act like money grows on trees. You're ungrateful."

"You're a slut. Your friends are whores."

"You're both useless and a disappointment."

"You've been stubborn and difficult since the day you were born."

"Why can't you do anything right? If you had, this never would have happened."

I believed everything she said, and I believed that it was my fault. The self-torture and guilt created an anger that settled in, got cozy, and stayed for years and years. I can't even say I was pissed. Pissed is an understatement. Pissed is a sugar-coated word with a cherry on top that didn't begin to describe how outraged I was at what my mother did to me. Driven by this anger, I set out to prove to her, to me, to someone—I don't know who, just anyone—that what she did was bad, and I was good. Once I proved it, I could put it all behind me and go on with my life.

In essence, I was competing with a ghost in an empty arena. Do you know how to declare victory in a battle with an unseen, unresponsive entity? What criteria do you use to determine the winner? Yeah, I don't know either. It was impossible to keep score. Yet every day I carried one tiny thought with me that impacted many of my choices. You probably passed right over that thought when you read it. Here it is again:

I was so outraged at what she did to me.

The thought *what she did to me* created feelings of turmoil, inadequacy, and worthlessness.

Mean Girl said, "How can you expect anyone to love or care about you after what your mother did to you? You weren't worth living for. You're so ugly, you got a face only a mother could love and she died so she wouldn't have to look at it no more."

I fought back and I fought hard. I was determined. I was going to be better than my mother. I was going to experience life. I was going to learn and grow and be happy. I seriously spent decades in active combat against my deceased mother. I was getting tired. The criteria I used to fight against my mother and compare myself to her wasn't making me any happier. I was learning and I was growing, but it wasn't working the way I had hoped it would.

Do you know what they call people who've spent as much time and money on their education and accumulated as many college credits as I have? They call them medical doctors. Except I'm not a medical doctor. After my mother's death, I set out to attend as many courses, workshops, and seminars as I could that offered some type of credential, or better yet, obtain as many degrees that I could. I will not bore you with the long laundry list of examples. I remember just before my mother died, she was taking evening classes. I'm not sure whether she was working toward a degree or just dabbling in things of interest. Either way, I believed every course I completed, every degree I obtained, every certificate with my name on it put my value further and further ahead of hers. I have a ton of education I didn't use or that didn't advance my career. Whenever I tried to justify why I wanted to chase down another credential I didn't need or wouldn't use, I came up empty. That's when I realized I was the lone participant in this competition I created in my head.

The more I learned, the more I discovered that I was too smart and too rational to continue the fight. It was consuming my life, my time, and my finances. I tried to quiet Mean Girl and convince her I was lovable and worth living for. Eventually, we reached a middle ground and agreed I would stop pursuing any additional education simply for the sake of trying to prove something to someone who doesn't exist.

Through all my learning and self-growth, I realized I was never responsible for what happened with my mother. But I was stuck in a negative thought loop for a long time. It works for you the same way it worked for me. First, we have a thought which leads to a feeling which causes a behavior that results in an outcome. This process goes round and round unless we change just one section of that loop. Once we do, it totally disrupts the spinning cycle. And that's where we can improve the outcome. We'll go more in-depth on this later.

Right now, the important thing to understand about this loop is the progression. Things that happen in our lives don't directly impact our feelings or our behavior. It's what we *think* about what's happening that creates the feeling that leads to our behavior. It was my mother's thoughts and feelings that led to my mother's action that caused her death. It was impossible that any of *my* behaviors caused my mother's death. My mother had her own loops that were controlled by her thoughts.

Once I understood and accepted that, I was able to release the regret and the guilt I had been carrying with me for most of my adult life. "I'm free!" I felt like Genie at the end of *Aladdin* when he's finally released from the lamp after ten thousand years. We all have our own loops, and our job is to work on our own thoughts, emotions, and behaviors.

What about my anger? How could I let go of it? I'd been holding on to it so close and tight for such a long time it was part of me. But, in all fairness, if I wasn't responsible for the thoughts that led to her actions, then her action wasn't responsible for my anger; my thoughts were. I started to consider different thoughts. Maybe this wasn't something she did to me. Maybe she wasn't thinking about me? Maybe she wasn't thinking at all. Maybe she did think about me, but she was going through too much. Maybe she hated leaving me. Maybe I'll never know. Maybe it just happened.

Author, coach, and motivational speaker Tony Robbins says suffering occurs when we are focused on ourselves, and we have the power to end our suffering through gratitude and serving others. After my mom died, my focus was solely on myself. I believed what she did was the direct cause of my guilt, anger, and feelings of inadequacy. I experienced a lot of suffering as a result. I believed I was a victim and there wasn't anything I could do about it. It changed my life when I finally realized I wasn't to blame for her thoughts, feelings, and actions, and she wasn't responsible for mine. Once that happened, I was able to shift my focus away from myself.

Changing what we think about the past or reprogramming an uncomfortable thought into something that serves us better is an available option. Believe me, I know it's hard, but it is possible.

In what ways are you holding on to the past?

Are you creating additional suffering by not letting go?

In what areas are your thoughts focused on yourself?

What can you do to end your suffering?

How can you show gratitude or serve others?

Next time you feel like you're suffering, notice where your thoughts are. It's totally normal to be thinking of yourself, especially when you experience heartache. Are you able to shift your focus a little? Maybe find something you're grateful for. A small sliver of a silver lining? Can you be of service to others? My mother was the second daughter my grandmother had lost since her husband died twenty years earlier. She was there to support me, but I don't remember who was there to support her. I didn't know it at the time, but looking back, I honestly think her service to others (me) helped her with her own sadness and suffering.

Earlier I said, "Maybe it was supposed to happen." I know, that probably seemed preposterous when you first read it. But I am who I am, just like you are who you are, because of our experiences. Maybe this is who we were supposed to become. I share my experiences with you in order to assure you that you've never done anything that left you unworthy of love.

Throughout this book, you'll find stories and techniques that will encourage you to let go of beliefs you've had your entire life so you can turn your Mean Girl around. It's a big step learning how to love, appreciate, and respect yourself regardless of your size, shape, or the amount of shit you've been through. But there's nothing that can keep you from embarking on that journey. I'll be here to guide you.

* * *

ACTIVITY:

In what ways are you holding on to the past?

Are you creating additional suffering by not letting go?

In what areas are your thoughts focused on yourself?

What can you do to end your suffering?

How can you show gratitude or serve others?

Next time you feel like you're suffering, notice where your thoughts are. It's totally normal to be thinking of yourself, especially when you experience heartache. Are you able to shift your focus a little? Maybe find something you're grateful for. A small sliver of a silver lining? Can you be of service to others?

❧ 3 ❧

MEAN GIRL LIE:

MY THOUGHTS ARE OUT OF CONTROL

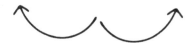

In the last chapter, I talked about how things that happen don't directly impact your feelings or your behavior. It's what you think about what happened that create the feelings that lead to your behavior.

This isn't an original concept. It's been used by other coaches like Tony Robbins and Brooke Castillo. It's a form of cognitive behavioral therapy (CBT) developed by Dr. Aaron Beck. CBT is based on the idea that how we think, feel, and act are all interrelated. This process is used in counseling and coaching to help clients gain control of the thoughts that create their emotions that lead to actions that create results (Thoughts > Emotions > Behavior > Outcome).

I've seen this presented before as a linear formula with the premise that when you change your thoughts then your emotions, actions, and outcomes naturally change. I agree. Where I disagree is suggesting you must focus solely on changing your thoughts. It can be too overwhelming or maybe even seem impossible to sit down and just change a thought. I believe you can implement change by intervening at any step in the progression by adjusting a thought, feeling, or action.

This process is often called a thought loop, but it consists of more than just thoughts orbiting inside your head. Part of the loop is inside your head—thoughts and feelings—but then the loop leaves your body for the behavior and outcome.

It's like an amusement park ride that starts in a tunnel, twists and turns a bit in the darkness, before spinning and flipping out into the open air and then curving around to end up back in the tunnel again. Nobody would call that a "tunnel ride," so I'm not sure why they call it a "thought loop."

I don't like it when things are confusing, so I try to make them as uncomplicated as possible, either by breaking them down into their simplest terms or by creating an analogy. Not just so it's easier to understand, but so it's also something you want to understand. You're going to find I do that a lot throughout this book. So I've broken down this CBT "thought loop" into something simpler. I'm calling my simplified version the Silver Lining Cycle. Why? Because you can make adjustments at any point in the cycle in a way that works best for finding a silver lining in a fact that you've attached a negative meaning to.

SO HOW DOES THIS SILVER LINING CYCLE WORK?

We start with a neutral fact. What you think, feel, and do as it pertains to that fact determines what you get. As you can see, I view it as circular rather than linear.

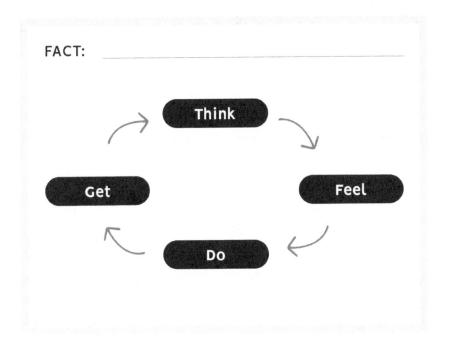

First there's a neutral FACT or situation. The cycle begins when something happens. Reality. Whatever it is, it's neutral. If people saw it or overheard it, they'd all agree, "It's a fact, Jack."

- The dog is barking.

- I ate pie.
- My sister did not eat pie.
- My co-worker is dieting.
- I overslept.
- It snowed seven inches.

None of these things have any meaning on their own. It's impossible to determine whether they are good or bad or neutral. It's what we think about them that gives them meaning. The FACT is the starting point of your Silver Lining Cycle. You can't change the facts (remember my fire?) You can only change what you think, feel, and do about it.

THINK

As soon as something happens, we attach meaning based on what we THINK about it. It'll either stay neutral or we'll view it as good or bad depending on the thought we attach to the fact. For example, let's use the fact that it snowed seven inches. If you don't live where it snowed and you don't know anyone who does, it'll likely remain neutral. Let's say Rex wants to go skiing. He sees the seven inches of snow as something good. Unlike Otis, who views the snow as a negative because it'll take him two hours to clear his ten-car driveway, and all he's got is a child-size toy shovel.

FEEL

Before we go any further, I want to note the term FEEL is being used to represent emotions such as *I feel sad* or *I feel happy*. It is not used to describe symptoms of how you are feeling physically. "I feel like I'm going to throw up." "It feels like I broke my toe." Now, back to the Silver Lining Cycle. How you FEEL is a result of what you THINK about what happened. Rex thinks the snow is great, so he's pretty happy about the seven inches. Otis, on the other hand, doesn't want to shovel, and he's feeling frustrated.

DO

What you DO depends on what you're thinking and feeling. Rex is doing a little happy dance and gathering his ski equipment and heading to the slopes. Otis is huffing around the house, banging things, and heading outside to shovel.

GET

What you GET is a result of what you do. Rex got to have fun hanging out with his friends while skiing. Otis froze his ass off using his four-year-old's toy shovel to clear the driveway. He did get a clean driveway to go along with his sore muscles. Notice how two people reacted differently to the same exact fact. For one, the fact was positive; for the other, the fact was negative.

THE SILVER LINING

Here's how we can change things around and turn the dark cloud into a silver lining. Remember, you can interrupt or make a change at any point in the cycle. Let's look at what Otis might do to change the cycle. Otis has hated snow his entire life. It would be impossible for him to just sit down and choose a new thought that would change how he feels and acts when it snows. What he can do, though, is ask himself, "What can I DO to help change what I think and feel about the snow?" This would interrupt the cycle with a new action. He could buy a larger shovel, a snowblower, a tractor, or hire a plow guy. That might change what he thinks and feels when he looks out the window and sees seven inches of snow.

TELL ME MORE ABOUT HOW TO MANIPULATE THE SILVER LINING CYCLE

Until you've done this for a while, it's hard to use the Silver Lining Cycle when you're deep in your own shit. For example, let's say just before you went out for the evening, you asked your husband to move the bedsheets from the washer into the dryer. When you get home at 10:00 p.m., you go to the dryer to get the clean sheets, and you find they're still sitting in the washing machine soaking wet. You're probably not going to ask yourself what you're going to think, feel, or do about this. You're probably going to lose your shit on him.

After you've experimented and played around with it a bit, it may become a little easier to ward off the immediate feelings of anger, but that's not to say you won't still get angry from time to time. We all do. Until then, it's easier to practice using this cycle after the fact, like a Monday morning quarterback. For example, after you fight with your husband and discover it didn't bring about a very good result, you can sit down and ask yourself what you could have thought, felt, or done differently so you wouldn't have ended up in such a huge battle.

Another way to practice using it is when you're dwelling on a situation that doesn't affect you as immediately as the dryer incident. Here are some examples.

Let's say the FACT is I don't have enough money to pay bills at the end of the month. You can start to work on the Silver Lining Cycle at the point of the result—the GET. Ask yourself, "What do I want to GET?" You might answer, "$1000 by the end of the month."

Now, you'd move on to the next step in the cycle—DO. You'd ask, "What do I need to DO to get $1000 by the end of the month?" One answer might be, "I can ask one hundred people to pay $10 for my autograph."

Next, you'd ask yourself, "How do I need to FEEL in order to get one hundred people to pay $10 for my autograph?" The answer, "I'd need to feel excited, motivated, and confident about getting this money and paying the bills."

What do I need to THINK about all this? Answer, "I'd be thinking about having the bills paid."

Let's try another one: This time the event or fact that happened is you got fired. Let's see how it plays out if we start with DO:

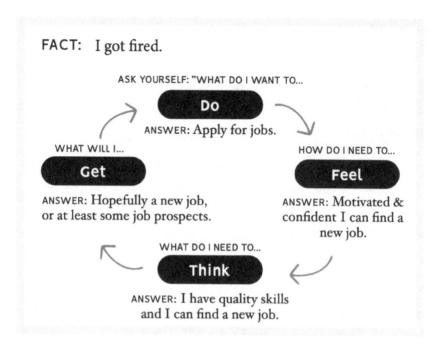

FACT: I got fired.

ASK YOURSELF: "WHAT DO I WANT TO...

Do

ANSWER: Apply for jobs.

WHAT WILL I...

Get

ANSWER: Hopefully a new job, or at least some job prospects.

HOW DO I NEED TO...

Feel

ANSWER: Motivated & confident I can find a new job.

WHAT DO I NEED TO...

Think

ANSWER: I have quality skills and I can find a new job.

Here's another example, starting with FEEL:

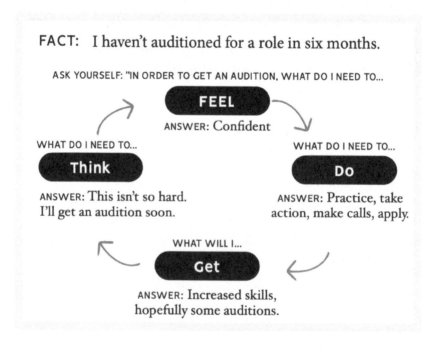

FACT: I haven't auditioned for a role in six months.

ASK YOURSELF: "IN ORDER TO GET AN AUDITION, WHAT DO I NEED TO...

FEEL

ANSWER: Confident

WHAT DO I NEED TO...

Think

ANSWER: This isn't so hard. I'll get an audition soon.

WHAT DO I NEED TO...

Do

ANSWER: Practice, take action, make calls, apply.

WHAT WILL I...

Get

ANSWER: Increased skills, hopefully some auditions.

In this example we start with THINK:

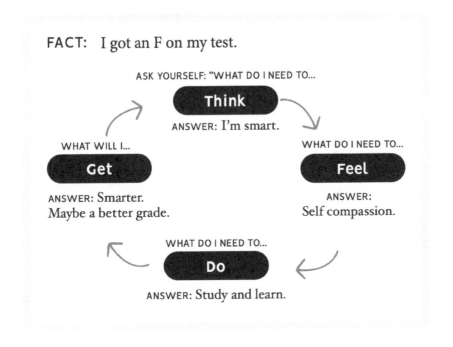

FACT: I got an F on my test.

ASK YOURSELF: "WHAT DO I NEED TO...
Think
ANSWER: I'm smart.

WHAT WILL I...
Get
ANSWER: Smarter.
Maybe a better grade.

WHAT DO I NEED TO...
Feel
ANSWER:
Self compassion.

WHAT DO I NEED TO...
Do
ANSWER: Study and learn.

Go to www.julieglynn.com for some worksheets to practice the Silver Lining Cycle yourself.

DISCREDIT YOUR THOUGHTS

It takes time and practice to go through the cycle as it's explained above. As I said, sometimes we're so deep in our own mess, we just want to scream and bang things. When that happens, we're not in a place to sit calmly and think rationally. The one area of the cycle we can quickly adjust is what we DO. Change the scenery, take a break, take a walk, read a book, or call a friend.

Changing what you do can also include gathering evidence or finding proof to "discredit" your thought. For example,

"I thought my boss was an ass until I sat next to him at the charity benefit."

"I didn't think I could run a 5K, but then I put my sneakers on and started running just a few minutes at a time."

"I thought for sure my appendix was rupturing then I looked online and saw it's located on the lower right side of the abdomen, and my ache was up near my left shoulder."

I was with my daughter when she was in labor. She repeatedly tried to convince us, "I can't do this." The evidence proved otherwise. If the nurse was in the room anytime my daughter groaned, "I can't do this," she immediately responded in a high-pitched nasally tone, "But you *are* doing it." That phrase has since become a joke in our family. And my daughter did, in fact, do it.

MEAN GIRL

I want to talk briefly about Mean Girl. She plays a really big part in your Silver Lining Cycle because she's the one putting thoughts into your head. (Remember, I'm personifying her so the thoughts in your head are easier to change.) The hope is that as we progress through the material in this book, Mean Girl will provide fewer critical, harsh, and unnecessary thoughts that require you to adjust your thinking with the Silver Lining Cycle. Of course, that's not to suggest we'll never attach an unnerving thought to a fact. The hope is that the combination of using the Silver Lining Cycle and calming Mean Girl will change what's going on in your head.

THE BLAME GAME

I want to reiterate something I said at the beginning of the chapter. It's what YOU think about what happens that create YOUR feelings that lead to YOUR actions (what YOU do). You're mistaken when you blame someone else for what you think, feel, or do. This blaming behavior starts in childhood and stays with some of us all the way through adulthood.

For example, little Wilma cries to the teacher, "Barney hurt my feelings. He said I'm stupid." Then the teacher brings Barney over, and they talk to him about how he needs to change what he says so Wilma doesn't get her feelings hurt.

"Wilma made me mad when she knocked over my blocks, so I said she was stupid."

Now we have to talk with Wilma about how she needs to act so she doesn't make Barney mad. No! Wilma is responsible for what she thinks, feels, and does. Barney is responsible for Barney. This lets both Wilma and Barney maintain their own power and control over their own thoughts, emotions, and behaviors.

Now that we've gone over the Silver Lining Cycle we'll be using in this book, let's go on and get to know more about Mean Girl.

❦ 4 ❦
MEAN GIRL LIE:

I'LL ALWAYS BE A VICTIM OF
MEAN GIRL

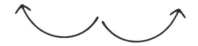

The other day I was talking with a friend who I know for a fact has a mean girl. She casually suggested maybe some people don't have one. I strongly disagreed. Right here from the beginning, I want to make it perfectly clear everyone has that voice in their head. You might recognize Mean Girl as someone who acts like this:

She causes you to question yourself and discourages you from taking risks.

She assumes strangers have idyllic lives, and you are a failure in comparison.

She judges the foods you eat and deprives your body of nourishment.

She convinces you your life will be perfect, and you'll fit in better if you're smaller.

She makes you doubt your intelligence or ability to succeed.

She keeps you from experiencing your feelings.

She convinces you you're not worthy of love, acceptance, or sexual pleasure.

She tells you it doesn't matter whether or not you try and give up; either way, you'll never measure up, and you'll be an embarrassment, a failure, or both.

She sabotages you with critical judgment.

She encourages poor choices and inflicts excessive guilt and self-doubt.

She's intimidating and scary.

Look back at this list. In spite of all this, you've spent years dragging Mean Girl along everywhere you go, believing every word she says. Who is this Mean Girl who puts you through hell? Believe it or not, she's that part of you whose job it is to keep you safe, help you avoid getting hurt, and make sure you survive. What? How can that be? I know, it doesn't make a bit of sense. We don't generally associate life-saving measures with criticism and harsh disapproval. But it's true.

So how is Mean Girl protecting you by jumping all over you as she does? She's been programmed based on a culture that primarily uses guilt, shame, and fear to foster positive change. We were raised hearing:

"Do this, or else!"

"Pick up your toys, or I'll throw them away."

"Stop crying, or I'll give you something to cry about."

"If you're good in the store you can have candy."

"Wipe that smile off your face, or I'll wipe it off for you."

"What were you thinking? You should be ashamed."

"Sit there until you've cleared your plate."

"Why can't you be more like your sister?"

"If don't finish you work you'll have to stay in and do it at recess."

Mean Girl is simply following a behavior modification method she's witnessed since her inception. She hangs on to everything she hears then echoes all the negative statements back at you. When my mother died and Mean Girl went on her rampage, she didn't concoct those accusations on her own. She was simply parroting criticism she'd heard directed at me in the past.

You've heard the saying there's safety in numbers? Mean Girl comes forward anytime she thinks you might separate from the crowd. She believes once you do, you're at risk. If you don't blend in, you're at risk. If you don't look like everyone else, you're at risk. If you don't behave like everyone else, you're at risk. As long as you're snuggled tightly within the safety of the masses, you're less likely to be a target.

Mean Girl came into existence as a defense mechanism to protect you and keep you safe. She presents as aggressive, hateful, and intimidating, keep in mind that's all she knows how to be. You have the upper hand. While she doesn't have the skills to deal with pain and heartache, you do. Without those skills of compassion, understanding, and forgiveness, she acts out. If you want her to be more compassionate with you, you need to be compassionate with her.

In order to fully love yourself, you have to accept that Mean Girl is a part of you. Throughout this book, I'm going to share different strategies you can use to give Mean Girl a makeover so she looks more like your friend than the scary old lady that lives in the run-down mansion at the end of the lane. It's not going to be easy, and it's going to require practice and patience. But you can do it.

Because she communicates harshly and uses scare tactics, naturally you'll want to reciprocate in kind. You'll want to go after her with the same level of disrespect. That won't work. Relationships don't heal through conflict. It only takes one rational person to change a relationship, and that's going to be you.

You'll need to increase your awareness of Mean Girl and her comments. You may need to continually notice and be aware of her for a while before you're ready to implement some strategies. For some of us, she's been hanging around calling the shots for so long, we're not quite ready to push her out of the driver's seat and slide her over to the passenger's side. Or even better yet, toss her into the backseat. You probably thought I was going to say toss her in the trunk, didn't you? The goal isn't that she's bound and gagged and locked away. The goal is to teach her to let go of the criticism and wisecracks and protect and keep you safe from a place of love and encouragement.

Let's get started.

MEAN GIRL LIE:

I'M FAT AND NOBODY LIKES ME

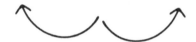

We talked about the Silver Lining Cycle. It's a simple formula we can manipulate to assure we live happily ever after. If you just think positively, feel happy, and do the right things, life would be perfect, and there'd be no reason for this book. Problem is, it's not that easy, and you've got Mean Girl with an endless flow of counterproductive thoughts constantly dripping into your head. It makes it almost impossible to change your thinking.

Remember Darlene? I mentioned her earlier? She's going to share stories from different points in her life in order to help you relate to this material and assure you that you are not alone.

When Darlene was in high school, her boyfriend, Clyde, worked nights as a cook at Buck's Burger Barn. Darlene was sure their puppy love was doggone perfect. She was so smitten she hardly even noticed the overpowering smell from the invisible grease cloud that surrounded him.

Every night, before she climbed into her ruffled canopy bed, she made sure her pink princess phone was on the nearby stand. No matter how late, Clyde called her as soon as he got home for a little bit of pillow talk. Often, she'd wake in the morning tangled in the phone cord having fallen asleep during their endearing nightly ritual. One night, things didn't go the way they typically did. She woke in the middle of the night to darkness and silence. She wasn't tangled in the phone cord. In fact, her phone was still sitting right there next to her bed where she'd placed it. No call? What could have happened? She couldn't call to check, not at this hour, she'd wake his entire family. Later the next day, when she finally did speak with Clyde, she learned he didn't even work the night before. What happened? Why hadn't he called? Why didn't they hang out? Instead of working, Clyde was on a date with that dainty girl Bonita who worked the counter at Buck's. Darlene was a wreck. How could this be happening? What happened to Darlene + Clyde = 4 Ever? Okay. Maybe forever was idealistic. She at least expected it to last longer than the brown paper bag book cover it was written on.

Mean Girl was pissed and she blamed Darlene.

"What did you expect? You're fat and ugly. Nobody likes you. You were lucky you even had a boyfriend!"

Mean Girl went on to accuse, "Of course Clyde is more interested in Bonita; she's smaller than you."

It's important to mention, at no time during this breakup was there ever any suggestion or evidence that Darlene's size or appearance had anything to do with Clyde's decision to start dating someone else. It was simply Darlene's thoughts about her body and the comparisons she made between herself and Bonita that created that fallacy in her head and the shit show that followed.

Mean Girl helped her create a plan. Darlene would take matters into her own hands. She could control this, and she was going to do just that. She'd get skinny, get her boyfriend back, and life would be perfect.

Darlene needed to act fast. Her happiness was at stake. She didn't exactly know how to diet, so she decided she simply wouldn't eat at all. It worked. In no time her weight loss was so noticeable, her track coach called her parents. They decided Darlene would have her body fat (or lack thereof) measured with those calibers that pinch your skin. She was underweight. As a result, her coach refused to let her compete or participate in practices until she stopped dieting and started gaining some weight. She was humiliated. Things weren't turning out at all how she'd hoped. The wrong people were paying attention. Clyde was long gone and had no idea she was lacking body fat. Wasn't that what he wanted? Wasn't that the key to their happiness? Darlene's plan turned out to be a huge fiasco. Things might have been different with a supportive voice in her head, but Darlene didn't have that. Mean Girl continued to bombard her with terrible allegations:

"You're a total screw up."

"You couldn't even do this right."

"You're worse off than you were before."

"Everyone at school thinks you're pathetic."

She felt so shitty, she just wanted to curl up and hide. The last thing she wanted to do was nourish her body. Mean Girl had filled Darlene's head with so many horrible thoughts. She didn't know what to do, and she certainly didn't know how to turn down the volume on Mean Girl.

Darlene was sure her happiness hinged on whether Clyde liked her or not. She also believed Mean Girl when she said being included, having friends, and being accepted by her peers were all based on the size of her body.

Darlene honestly believed if she could just change what was happening around her, she'd be happy. She thought she could do that by changing the size of her body. No wonder she was so miserable. She was chasing the clouds. She had no idea how to control her thoughts or how to look inside herself for the happiness she was seeking.

I want to pause here and reiterate Darlene was a teenager in high school. Learning how to do this is complicated and requires practice and guidance. Darlene didn't have either. She did an excellent job of hiding her unhealthy thoughts and feelings about her body, which often start in adolescents, from anyone who might have been willing to help her.

Darlene didn't know how to look inside herself for happiness, and even if she did, she didn't want to. It seemed so much easier if Clyde would just change his mind then she'd be happy again. It doesn't work like that. Darlene has to do the work herself and take charge of creating her own happiness. Don't get me wrong. Darlene was putting in a lot of effort changing her body. She thought if she changed her size, it would change the facts. She should have put that energy toward changing her thinking. Darlene's plan left her power-less and it put Clyde in charge of her happiness. He certainly wasn't doing a very good job at that.

Unfortunately, she can't change the facts. In this situation, the fact is Clyde broke up with Darlene. She didn't like how that made her think or feel, so she decided to focus on her actions rather than her thoughts. It looked like this:

FACT: Clyde broke up with Darlene

Think

Clyde doesn't like me
because I'm fat

Feel

Rejected

Get

1. Suspended from track
2. Attention from parents & coach

Do

Diet & change her size

If she'd had the maturity and guidance, she could have asked herself, "How do I want to feel?" The answer to that question could have been any of the following: happy, confident, included. The next question she would have asked is, "What do I need to think in order to feel happy?" or "What can I do to feel happy and confident?"

She could have thought, "If Clyde doesn't want to hang out with me, then it's good we broke up. Why would I want to spend time with someone who doesn't want to be around me?"

She could have thought, "Perhaps he has more in common with Bonita than he has with me."

She could've even thought, "I deserve someone better than Clyde. He didn't even break up with me before he started dating again."

Finally, she could've thought, "Maybe this was supposed to happen."

All these suggestions are higher order thinking skills which, again, would have been difficult for someone Darlene's age. To be quite honest, regardless of her age, she could very well have been so deep in her sadness and pain that she couldn't find any silver linings from the cycle. Not right now, anyway. Sometimes it takes a while before we find a silver lining. That's okay.

When that happens, try to find a silver lining somewhere else. Your brain can't hold space for two opposing thoughts at the same time. In other words, you can't feel bad and feel good at the same time. If you are stuck and can't find a silver lining in your current situation, look around and find something good to focus on from somewhere else. Darlene could find some silver linings (positive things) that have nothing to do with the shit storm she was in the middle of. So can you. I know it's not easy finding a bunch of positives when you're experiencing extreme discomfort. Let me help.

I want you to take out a sheet of paper and make a list of positive things in your life. If you're struggling to come up with something positive, consider including things like, "I have the ability to hold this book and read it." What else can you think of? Keep adding to the list as you come up with more ideas. Refer to this list whenever you're having a hard time and don't see a silver lining.

MEAN GIRL

Darlene was rejected when Clyde broke up with her. This created fear for Mean Girl because Darlene was at risk. She would no longer blend in and could possibly be ostracized from the group. Mean Girl created fear, and Darlene panicked along with her even though none of those things were even remotely possible. Darlene got her heart broken, and she and Mean Girl both experienced the pain and neither of them knew how to handle it. In order to eliminate unnecessary discomfort, it's important to pacify Mean Girl as soon as we can.

THE FIRST STEP TO SUBDUE MEAN GIRL

We usually refer to people in positions of authority with some level of formality. Dr. Feelgood or Professor Hardgrade. When I was hanging out with my friends in high school, we'd refer to our teachers and parents by their first names. Of course, never to their face. We felt like we were on a more level playing field when we'd ask, "Do you think Ed and Nadine will let you use their car on Saturday night?"

"So what did Art and Judy think of your new boyfriend?"

"Can you believe Marge gave me a C- on my research paper?"

When we're on a first-name basis, it suggests familiarity, mutual respect, and equal distribution of power. You can take away any implied authority Mean Girl has and create a balance between the two of you by giving her a name. Choose anything you want. Make it fun. Pick something that gives you a good vibe. A name that you can respect and care for. What name feels appropriate? We're going to work a lot more on reprogramming Mean Girl, but in the meantime, give her a name. It will put the two of you on a more level playing field.

We've talked about two important topics here and really need to distinguish that each are separate issues. One is the Silver Lining Cycle and how we can learn to manipulate it, so we don't feel horrible like Darlene did. Let me quickly recap.

Remember, when you don't like how you're feeling, you can choose to change what you THINK, what you FEEL, or what you DO. Ask yourself, "How do I want to think or feel?" and/or "What can I do?"

It takes a lot of practice before you can do it automatically, but eventually you'll get the hang of it.

The second topic is the issue of reprogramming Mean Girl. She freaked out when Clyde rejected Darlene. By naming her, Darlene is better equipped to defuse similar situations when they arrive. What both of these processes have in common is they take some practice. But don't worry. Soon you'll be using both of them to your advantage.

ACTIVITY:

Make a list of positive things in your life. If you're struggling to come up with something positive, consider including things like, "I have the ability to hold this book and read it."

What else can you think of? Keep adding to the list as you come up with more ideas. Refer to this list whenever you're having a hard time and don't see a silver lining.

MEAN GIRL STRATEGY:

Give Mean Girl a name. Choose anything you want. Make it fun. Pick something that gives you a good vibe. A name that you can respect and care for. What name feels appropriate and why?

❧ 6 ❧

MEAN GIRL LIE:

I'LL NEVER MEASURE UP

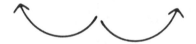

Like many of us, Darlene used to be both obsessed with and controlled by her bathroom scale. She has since tucked it away under the bed and no longer uses it as a tool to measure her worth. Instead, she uses it every now and then to weigh her luggage right before a trip.

During the years her life was dictated by diets and exercise, she was constantly searching for some external validation of her worth. She never believed she was small enough, good enough, or deserving enough. The minute she opened her eyes in the morning, Mean Girl immediately recapped everything she had eaten the previous day and compared it to how much she had exercised. This daily self-torture helped prepare her for what she could expect to see when she got on the scale. The number she saw meant everything. It was the criterion she used to determine if it was going to be a good day or a bad day. Depending on the number, she'd decide if she would eat today or starve herself in revenge for her body refusing to shed fat. If she was going to go through this daily diet hell obsessing, starving, and sacrificing, she damn well better be losing weight.

Most importantly, Mean Girl had an irrational belief that if the scale's number was within the range that society—or the $72-billion weight loss industry—deemed ideal for her height, then her life would be perfect.

When Darlene got up, she'd go to the bathroom, strip down, and get on the scale. If the scale showed a smaller number than the last time she stood on it, she was encouraged. She was heading in the right direction. But oh no! If the number was the same, or heaven forbid, even an ounce higher, she was devastated. All that work and she wasn't getting any closer to the perfect life she was sure she'd find just on the other side of weight loss.

Regardless of what she saw, most days she did a do-over. She'd put her pajamas back on, climb back into bed with her phone, check email, check Facebook, or play a game. After a little while, without having anything to eat or drink, she'd jump up and follow the exact same routine. Just in case she'd missed something, she'd recap everything she'd eaten the day before and compare it again to how much she'd exercised. She'd go to the bathroom, strip down, and hop on the scale, hoping this time for a smaller number. Sometimes she would repeat this cycle three or four times before she'd finally get up, get dressed, and begin her day.

That may seem a bit obsessive and unnecessary, but it never ended. Several times throughout the day, Darlene would get back on the scale, still longing to see the decrease that would increase her value. If she went to the bathroom, she'd get on the scale. Clipped her nails, get on the scale. Move her body, get on the scale. Blow her nose, get on the scale. Get a haircut, get on the scale. Before bed, get on the scale. Get up at night, get on the scale.

Intellectually she knew if the number went down, it wasn't necessarily an indication of fat loss. Yet she couldn't apply the same logical thinking if the number went up. She wouldn't consider the possibility that a higher number didn't necessarily mean she'd gained fat even though there are a number of reasons her weight might fluctuate throughout the day. The two that are most relevant to Darlene are the amount of water she drank and whether or not she had done any exercise.

What I've described is Darlene's morning routine after a day of strict dieting and exercising. If she had failed to follow the rules the day before, it was like waking up at the gates of hell. Mean Girl harped on her for whatever indulgence or weakness she had given in to the previous day.

She'd attack her character. "You're weak and you don't have any willpower."

She'd belittle her by telling her, "You should've tried harder."

She'd guilt trip Darlene by saying, "If only you had exercised more."

She'd threaten her with things like, "Your life will never be perfect. You deserve to be miserable."

And Mean Girl would condemn Darlene's entire existence saying things like, "You're a horrible person."

Darlene felt so guilty and ashamed. Why? She hadn't cheated anyone. She didn't lie. She wasn't a criminal. She didn't wake up in a jail cell or on the run in a cheap rundown motel room. She had nothing to feel guilty about. She ate some food.

Darlene's not alone. I know she's not. I know too many people, myself included, who've woken up with the same intense regret. We'd just enjoyed some food. But there was a price to pay for that number on the scale.

There's an emotional "cost-benefit ratio" we forget to consider every time we get on the scale. How are you going to feel about it? What are you going to get from it? Remember, the number is neutral. It's the fact in the cycle. It's the thoughts you attach to that number that gives it meaning. Is it worth it? Sometimes ignorance is bliss. Take yourself through a hypothetical cycle and consider the different possible outcomes, then ask yourself, "Is it worth it?"

The scale in no way whatsoever measures anyone's worth as a person. There's no reason to feel guilty for nourishing your body. There's no reason to attach meaning to what you see when you stand on the scale. Your perfect life is not contingent on the scale.

One Monday morning, Darlene experienced so much excitement one would've thought she had won the lottery. In her mind, it was far better than a million-dollar jackpot. She'd lost eight pounds. Overnight. Just like that. All her troubles magically disappeared, and her world was glorious and filled with rainbows and unicorns. Until the next morning. Absent any consideration the eight-pound decrease might be a fluke, she jumped out of bed and tore off her clothes as she raced into the bathroom hoping to see another eight-pound drop. It didn't happen. She didn't lose any weight. In fact, she gained eight pounds. So, Tuesday morning she weighed exactly the same as she did on Sunday morning. Suddenly dark clouds rolled in, the rainbow faded away, and a vicious windstorm blew the unicorn off into the distance, never to be seen again, leaving behind the same person she was just two short days ago. Except she was so deflated and angry, she was actually worse off than she was on Sunday.

She never determined why her scale showed the eight-pound loss. It actually doesn't matter. What we do know is nothing about Darlene changed except her thoughts about her value as a person, based solely on the number she saw on the scale.

Darlene had always struggled with self-confidence. She'd been working on strategies with her coach for a while, but she was skeptical. She still doubted she had unique value as a person in any size body. With some coaching and reflection, she recognized the absurdity in her twenty-four-hour ride on the emotional roller coaster. It was the jolt she needed to help shift her perspective. She was ready to give up the inconsistent emotions she experienced every time she stood on the scale. When she looked back, she couldn't believe she thought she had lost eight pounds overnight; well, she kind of believed it because she'd wished for it for so long. What she really couldn't believe was the level of excitement she felt when she believed it was true. She also couldn't believe she honestly thought her worth had increased because she'd lost eight pounds. She'd heard it a number of times, but this experience solidified the fact that she was still the same person regardless of the number on the scale. She knew she didn't want to experience those emotional highs and lows anymore, so she decided she was ready to start examining her obsessive scale behavior. She didn't enjoy waking up every single day to immediate disappointment and emotional turmoil. So, she started working on a new morning routine.

These are some of the things Darlene considered implementing into her new morning routine.

When she opens her eyes to the gift of another day, she accepts it with gratitude.

She gets ready for her day by listening to a playlist of feel-good songs.

She takes note of all the things she's grateful for: her warm bed, her family, her health, her career, and her cat.

She journals or reads quotes or stories intended to create a positive start to the day.

She observes the beauty of nature, the trees, the sky, and the animals she sees outside her window.

In a dream world, Darlene would toss that scale out and do all these things the very next day, but that's not realistic. She still thinks about what she ate. She's still curious about her weight. She just doesn't let those things consume her thinking. Some days she implements something from the list above. Some days she just gets up, goes to the bathroom, and heads to the kitchen. Some days she lies in bed on the computer. The point isn't to do a complete turn-around overnight. Growth happens slowly over time. What's important is that Darlene has some tools at hand to help her shift from her obsessive scale behavior to something that better serves her.

We're going to talk a lot about self-compassion. One of the best forms of self-compassion is to ensure you start your day off on a positive note. That's why it was so instrumental that Darlene was willing to shift her morning routine. I invite you to stop here and take a minute to create a list of things you might do in the morning to ensure you get started on the right foot. Simply jot thoughts down as they come to you. Don't worry about perfect sentences, grammar, or punctuation. Tomorrow morning or within the next few days, pick one of these things and experiment with it. What did you discover?

In addition to the number on the scale, Mean Girl uses all sorts of other numbers to judge us. She uses tape measures, clothing sizes, grades, carats, financial statements, salaries, age, square footage, friends, or price tags to either make us feel like crap or artificially inflated.

Why do we do this when we know numbers don't indicate our value as a person? Mean Girl creates these thoughts then gives meaning to our numbers. We think certain numbers ensure we'll have a perfect life. Ask yourself, "What are you making these numbers mean?" Let me illustrate an example of this using the cycle.

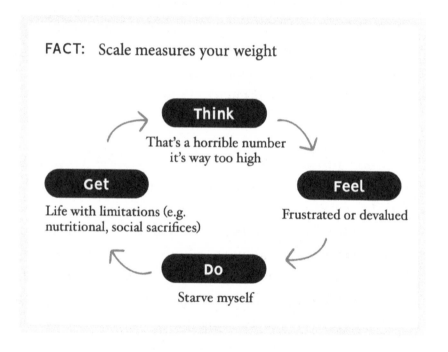

FACT: Scale measures your weight

Think
That's a horrible number
it's way too high

Feel
Frustrated or devalued

Do
Starve myself

Get
Life with limitations (e.g.
nutritional, social sacrifices)

Here's an example of a different loop with the same FACT—the scale measures your weight.

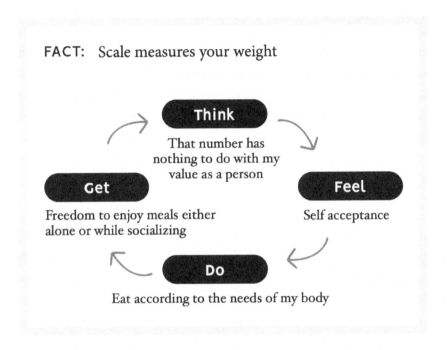

FACT: Scale measures your weight

Think — That number has nothing to do with my value as a person

Feel — Self acceptance

Do — Eat according to the needs of my body

Get — Freedom to enjoy meals either alone or while socializing

I encourage you to fill in your own cycle. Start with the fact—the scale measures your weight. Now, fill in the think, feel, do, and get sections as they apply to you. Visit www. julieglynn.com for a worksheet to help you do this very thing.

It's been said that every day you wake up means you still have a purpose here on earth. As long as you have a purpose, whether you know what it is or not, you have value. A value that's not contingent on size, success, achievement, or appearance. Earlier I told you about my obsession with academic credentials. Take it from me, degrees and certificates don't equal self-worth or self-acceptance. Take out a sheet of paper and make a list of everywhere you add value. This may be very hard to do. I'm going to walk you through it. As I said above, just the fact you are living and breathing is a sign you have value. First, you have to trust and accept that. Can you do that? My wish for you is that you're in a place where you can easily spout off a few obvious signs of your value. In the event you're not in that space, use baby steps to get there. For example, I want you to consider something like this: if you ever eat at a restaurant, you have value to the wait staff. They get paid to serve you. If you weren't there, they might get sent home, or worse yet, not have a job at all. If you have a car, you are valuable to the people who work in the factories making those cars, the mechanics who repair and inspect cars, and the people who work at the store where you get gas. Again, don't worry about sentence structure, grammar, or punctuation. Just get your ideas on paper. The more you think about this, the more things will come up. Tell Mean Girl, "MG" (the name you gave her), please go find some evidence I have value." Then let her get to work. She'll pop ideas into your head when you're not expecting it.

Back to Mean Girl. She might be mean, and she may be a little unconventional in her methods, but she's not a total dim wit. She's just tangled in the fear-mongering net the media and the $72-billion weight loss industry cast over us. They tell us how we need to look in order to fit it. Mean Girl is afraid you'll be slaughtered if you don't fit the mold they use to define beauty. She has no idea she was deceived. But then, how could she? You probably didn't either.

This is an opportunity to bond with Mean Girl. There's an ancient proverb that says, "The enemy of my enemy is my friend." That means two parties should work together against a common enemy. That would be you and Mean Girl against the weight loss industry that's out to make money on you hating your body.

Take Mean Girl's hand and work together to break away from the belief that media, society, and scales define beauty. You were both duped, and you can support each other. Remember, when you hurt, Mean Girl hurts. When you feel at ease, she feels at ease. There's no reason you can't have conversations with Mean Girl just like you would with one of your friends. That is the goal, by the way. Start by sharing your frustration of falling into the weight loss industry's trap then celebrate breaking free from it. I encourage you to try this. Have a conversation with her and see what happens. Tell her, "I'm so glad we're no longer brainwashed and will never spend another dime supporting the industry that spent so many years deceiving us."

Share your excitement with her and tell her, "We can enjoy doing so many things now that we're free." In the beginning, there may be some regretful thoughts. But there's no reason to look backward. While you still have her hand in yours, turn around and face forward and enjoy your common bond.

ACTIVITY:

Create a list of things you might do in the morning to ensure you get started on the right foot. Simply jot thoughts down as they come to you. Don't worry about perfect sentences, grammar, or punctuation. Tomorrow morning or within the next few days, pick one of these things and experiment with it. What did you discover?

Take out a sheet of paper and make a list of everywhere you add value. This may be very hard to do. I'm going to walk you through it. As I said above, just the fact you are living and breathing is a sign you have value. First, you have to trust and accept that. Can you do that? My wish for you is that you're in a place where you can easily spout off a few obvious signs of your value. In the event you're not in that space, use baby steps to get there. For example, I want you to consider something like this: if you ever eat at a restaurant, you have value to the wait staff. They get paid to serve you. If you weren't there, they might get sent home, or worse yet, not have a job at all. If you have a car, you are valuable to the people who work in the factories making those cars.

MEAN GIRL STRATEGY:

Take Mean Girl's hand and bond with her and work together as common enemies. Send her off to do some errands, like you did when you made the list of your value and told her, "Go find evidence of my value." Ask her for evidence or answers then release it and let her be while she goes off to find it.

Start conversations with her just like you would a friend. Share your frustration of falling into the weight loss industry's trap then celebrate breaking free from it. Have a conversation with her and see what happens. Tell her, "I'm so glad we're no longer brainwashed and will never spend another dime supporting the industry that spent so many years deceiving us."

Share your excitement with her and tell her, "We can enjoy doing so many things now that we're free." In the beginning, there may be some regretful thoughts. But there's no reason to look backward. While you still have her hand in yours, turn around and face forward and enjoy your common bond.

❦ 7 ❧
MEAN GIRL LIE:

I'M NOT AS GOOD AS EVERYONE ELSE

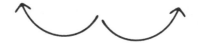

When we compare ourselves to ideas we create in our head about other people, we often come out feeling like a failure. We imagine people are living the perfect life we've always dreamed of, then we feel disappointed with our lives. Many of us can probably relate to how that happened with Darlene.

She watched from her window as her new neighbor moved in. Every day, all summer, as she spied on the neighbor coming and going, Mean Girl cast judgment causing Darlene to feel intimidated. Mean Girl thought the neighbor looked like the refined New York City penthouse type with flawless skin and long, thick flowing hair. She had perfectly manicured nails, bright white teeth, and not an ounce of fat on a body dressed in fashionable clothing, shoes, and handbags. Surely anyone as stunning as she must have a lot of money, an amazing career, overflowing confidence, tons of friends, and influence. Mean Girl chastised Darlene about her frumpy appearance, her mediocre lifestyle, and her modest home and furnishings. Darlene yearned for the extravagant, luxurious life she assumed the neighbor had.

Everyone had met the newcomer, Peyton, except Darlene. Darlene had no intention of ever meeting her. Mean Girl encouraged her not to like Peyton based on the little snippets she'd gathered from looking at her through the window. What's really messed up is Darlene was so brainwashed by Mean Girl, she didn't see how her thoughts about Peyton were unfair and unhealthy. Darlene would be outraged if she ever suspected someone else was judging another person based on appearance. But here she was, letting Mean Girl convince her to do just that.

One fall morning, Peyton came outside just as Darlene was starting her morning walk. Before Darlene could escape, Peyton introduced herself and asked if she could join her. The last thing Darlene wanted to do was walk with Peyton, but she was unable to come up with a viable excuse fast enough, so she reluctantly agreed.

From the minute they took their first step, Peyton started talking and rambled nonstop. She dominated the entire walk with a conversation that lacked the sophistication and depth Darlene expected. Peyton spoke mostly using slang terms and a great deal of vulgarity. Darlene was both surprised and impressed. They had just met, yet Peyton felt comfortable enough to simply be herself. But it didn't stop there. Peyton completely pulled back the curtain and opened up to Darlene. Peyton said she was envious of Darlene as she appeared to have a loving caring relationship with her husband, Stew. Then she went on to share her horrible history with men. Throughout high school and college, she dated men who just wanted sex then dumped her once they got it. Eventually, she dropped out of college and got a high-paying job as a live-in nanny where she had a six-year affair with the father of the children. Finally, his wife discovered it and kicked her out, ending both the affair and her nanny job at the same time. Desperate for money and a place to live, she quickly hooked up with a much older man and soon became his fifth wife. That led Peyton to grumble about how badly he and his adult children treated her, causing her to distance herself and lose all contact with her friends and family. She described how the stepchildren incessantly accused her of fraud and infidelity until the relationship inevitably broke down and recently ended in divorce. If it wasn't for the small financial settlement she received from that marriage, she'd be destitute without any job skills or savings to support herself and her lifestyle. She claimed she was going to run out of money soon, and she didn't know what she was going to do. The thought of not keeping up her gym membership was terrifying. What would she do with herself those twenty hours a week she spent at the gym? Darlene could sense the exhaustion in her voice as Peyton described the amount of time and money she spent maintaining her appearance.

Darlene was speechless throughout their entire walk. Not that she could've gotten a word in edgewise. All she could think was, "How could someone as pretty and well put together as Peyton be such a hot mess?" Secondly, "How could Peyton possibly be envious of me?" Darlene wondered.

It turns out, Peyton was a very sweet, authentic person who was willing to open up and connect with others. Darlene was ashamed of herself for the assumptions she had made. Mean Girl did a complete 180 degree turn and blamed Darlene. She hissed, "How could you be so judgmental? You should be ashamed and embarrassed." Then she confirmed, "You are a horrible person. Peyton should be the one who hates you, not the other way around."

Darlene's walk with Peyton was very eye-opening. She discovered that there wasn't a doubt in her mind she'd much rather have her life and her ass exactly the way they were than Peyton's life and her cute little butt. Which led Darlene to the realization that she'd made two significant errors.

First, she'd made inaccurate assumptions about Peyton, and second, she'd avoided Peyton based on those assumptions. Neither one of these served Darlene. She realized that for months she made herself miserable because of the thoughts Mean Girl filled her head with about someone else's appearance. Once she discovered her error, she felt just as bad at how she'd acted.

You can save yourself this agony. I know it's hard, but it serves no purpose comparing yourself to others. The silver lining in this situation was that Darlene had the opportunity to discover the truth about Peyton, and once she did, she discovered something about herself too.

Some people never get the opportunity to peek behind the curtain, and they carry these uncorroborated feelings of inadequacy and animosity forever.

ISN'T THE PURPOSE OF MEAN GIRL TO KEEP US SAFE AND SECURE?

This doesn't make any sense. Darlene was safe and secure at home looking out her window while Mean Girl made these inaccurate assumptions about Peyton. How is Mean Girl keeping her safe when she's filling her head with lies, exaggerations, and assumptions?

Mean Girl uses whatever method she can to keep us from becoming an outlier. In this situation, Mean Girl feared Darlene was too run-of-the-mill for someone like Peyton, and that put her at risk. Mean Girl thought if she used scare tactics to intimidate Darlene to stay away from Peyton, it would protect her from the same unsubstantiated judgment from Peyton that would cause Darlene pain and rejection.

But we are the ones who get to decide the criteria we use to determine whether or not we fit in or whether or not we are at risk. We decide whether or not we want to grow and change. We don't have to give Mean Girl the power to make that decision for us the way Darlene did.

HOW DO WE DO THIS?

Become okay with yourself and conscious of the fact that from time to time, everyone experiences the same unpleasant emotions you do. Notice I said to become "okay"? Of course, the goal is to love yourself. But that's a tall order, so let's start with becoming okay.

There's a misconception that anyone who fits within the mold of society or the media's definition of beauty has a perfect life. Nobody has a perfect life because nobody experiences happiness all the time. Sometimes we experience positive emotions, sometimes we experience negative emotions, and sometimes we're just neutral.

I know sometimes it feels like you got all the unpleasant experiences, and someone else got all the pleasant ones. That's simply not true, but it can feel unfair and frustrating and create an even stronger desire to compare when you believe that. We all experience a split of positive, negative, and neutral emotions; it's just that we don't always notice when things are going well. But we sure do notice when things are a mess. Try to start noticing when you feel positive or neutral, and you'll see there is a balance.

HOW DO WE BECOME OKAY WITH OURSELVES?

Decrease comparison and increase compassion. Open your awareness to the fact that everyone experiences discomfort from time to time. Try setting aside comparison and leaning in toward compassion.

After Darlene discovered Peyton had lovable qualities and her assumptions about her were incorrect, she immediately felt compassion toward Peyton but felt loathing toward herself for being so judgmental. Darlene can turn the compassion she feels toward Peyton around toward herself. She too has the same lovable qualities and deserves the same level of compassion she's now feeling toward Peyton. She just made a mistake.

Also, choose thoughts and feelings that best serve you. Where are you making comparisons that leave you feeling insignificant? What can you do to challenge your thinking? What can you think instead that will improve how you feel about yourself?

When you see someone and you THINK, "She's pretty." How do you want to FEEL about that? Depending on how you feel, it's going to impact what you DO. Use experiences like Darlene's to help guide your choices in the future.

Let's look at how the Silver Lining Cycle worked in this situation for Darlene.

The FACT is Darlene has a new neighbor.

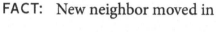

FACT: New neighbor moved in

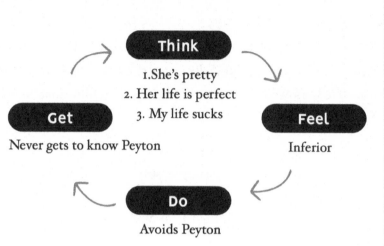

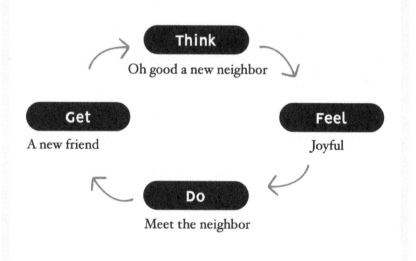

The second cycle's gotta feel way better than what Darlene went through with the first cycle.

THAT'S NOT SO EASY WITH MEAN GIRL

When you get sucked in by Mean Girl like Darlene did making judgments or comparisons, forgive yourself. When you make a mistake, forgive yourself. You have nothing to gain by beating yourself up and everything to gain by offering yourself forgiveness.

When Mean Girl provokes unpleasant thoughts, be aware of her. Try to appreciate that she's doing the best she can. We're not always in imminent danger when she comes to our rescue. Sometimes she's just acting on what she perceives as a possible threat. Understand when we fail, Mean Girl fails. When we hurt, Mean Girl hurts. Sometimes she's so scared and confused she doesn't know what to do. Offer her some reassurance. Call her by the name you've given her and tell her, "We're going to be okay." It's okay if you think someone is pretty. It's okay if you think someone has way more money than you have. These are all just thoughts.

When I was younger, my friend and I loved to make up songs. We'd sing them ad nauseam until everyone in our family would yell at us to stop. How do we soothe babies? With lullabies. This is such a fun Mean Girl strategy. You can make up your own songs. Here are a few lines of a lullaby I recrafted to give you an idea of how fun this can be.

Hush little Mean Girl, don't say a word.

You're only repeating what you've heard.

Soon everything will be changing,

Talk to me nicely, and I'll stop singing.

* * *

ACTIVITY:

Where are you making comparisons that leave you feeling insignificant? What can you do to challenge your thinking? What can you think instead that will improve how you feel about yourself?

MEAN GIRL STRATEGY:

Make up your own songs to sing to her. Here are a few lines of a lullaby I recrafted to give you an idea of how fun this can be.

Hush little Mean Girl, don't say a word.

You're only repeating what you've heard.

Soon everything will be changing,

Talk to me nicely, and I'll stop singing.

❈ 8 ❈

IF EVERYONE ELSE GOT THEIR SHIT TOGETHER I COULD BE HAPPY

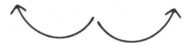

While I was writing this book, I questioned whether or not I was expected to put a quote at the beginning of every chapter. I did not want to do that. I was excited when I found out it wasn't necessary. With that being said, I'm going to put a quote at the beginning of this chapter. I know, it's just extra words, and personally, I never read those quotes. But this one is important and meaningful. I need you to have this at the forefront of your thinking as you read this chapter. It's by Eleanor Roosevelt,

No one can make you feel inferior without your consent.

Wouldn't it be great if people behaved in such a way that we found everything they said and did pleasing? It would be such a wonderful dream world to live in. A place where we never experience discomfort or stress. It would be everyone else's responsibility to make sure things are always delightful for us. That will never happen. Unfortunately, some people spend most of their life believing their happiness is a direct result of other people's behavior. Darlene was one of those people.

Darlene would get really worked up and upset anytime someone made a comment or voiced an opposing opinion about food, diet, body size, or weight. She placed blame on anyone who made these types of comments. How dare they victimize her like that? She called these incidents or comments "triggers," and once she was triggered, she considered herself no longer responsible for what she thought, felt, or did. It was the one who made the statements who was at fault.

It's probably important to dive a little deeper here into what "triggers" are. Triggers are generally used to describe events or statements that cause intense emotions or spark memories of past trauma. Recently, the term has become more broadly used to describe any unwelcome comment that creates uneasy thoughts or feelings.

Here's an example of how I was recently triggered. We had a contained immediately extinguished fire in our oven less than two months after we moved back into our house after experiencing a fire just a year before. I don't mean something overcooked causing every smoke alarm in the house to go off. I mean the flames inside the oven were at least six inches high.

The house was filling with smoke. I totally lost it. I cried and I didn't want to stop. Seeing the smoke and the flames, as harmless as they turned out to be, triggered the same emotions I'd had a year ago when we lost everything in a fire. I felt the same excruciating pain in my chest and stomach that I'd had a year ago. I could feel my heart racing in my chest. I felt an immediate fear of emptiness and loss. The same emptiness and loss I'd had just experienced throughout the previous year. I was scared. I don't want to go through that again.

If you have suffered a traumatic experience, let me remind you, this book is not intended to deal with related issues such as PTSD. Additionally, this book is not meant to treat eating disorders. If you are experiencing intense feelings or trauma or an eating disorder, you should seek the assistance of a professional. If you are working to improve your life by changing your thought patterns, keep reading.

Because Darlene was searching for a world where other people made her comfortable, secure, and happy, she, like many others, resorted to blaming others for being "triggered" instead of calling it what it really is: "uncomfortable," "attacked," "offended," or "hurt." We all have things that can provoke unpleasant thoughts or memories. If Darlene feels self-conscious or inadequate because of what someone says to her, that's different from getting triggered to relive past trauma. There's a psychological difference between "triggers" and "hurt feelings." For the sake of this book and this chapter, regardless of what you call it, as Eleanor Roosevelt said, "No one can make you feel inferior without your consent."

Nobody can hurt Darlene's feelings. Her own thoughts create her feelings.

Darlene belonged to a virtual body acceptance group. Members of the group shared stories about being "triggered" by what other people think, feel, and do. They'd get angry together and complain, "How could someone smaller and prettier than I am dare say she isn't satisfied with her appearance? Doesn't she know how triggering that is to someone less attractive?"

They'd all sympathize and coddle each other. They'd virtually handhold and pat each other's back. Then they'd encourage one another to confront these intentional haters who triggered them and caused them to feel so bad about themselves.

The unwritten motto was that people needed to stop triggering them. They made it their mission to change everyone who did or said something to cause their insecure feelings. Darlene didn't realize at the time, but the members of her group believed that taking back their control and caring for themselves meant making others feel as bad as they felt from being "triggered."

If they couldn't force these people to change, then ultimately, they would unfriend them and remove them from their lives. That'll teach them to have their own thoughts. Darlene was in. She felt so empowered. Unfortunately, Darlene's participation in this group had her so deep in victim mentality, she was just looking for a reason to snap. That's exactly what she did.

Shortly after her family finished eating Thanksgiving dinner, Darlene's mom brought out dessert. She went around the table asking what everyone wanted then served them. Darlene had already eaten half of a piece of pie by the time her mom got around to her sister Mellie who declined dessert and commented, "Nothing for me, I want to look good in my bathing suit next month when Jack and I go on vacation."

Mean Girl taunted,

"Oh no she didn't."

"Did she just say what I think she said?"

"Did you hear that?"

"Your sister has more willpower than you."

"You lack discipline."

"She thinks you're fat and shouldn't eat pie."

Darlene ignored Mean Girl.

Darlene's other sister Louisa jumped in and suggested Mellie try this new diet pill she'd recently started using. She wasn't having any trouble passing up desserts since she started taking it, as it made anything with sugar in it taste like raw sewage.

That was it! Darlene tossed her napkin onto the table. She refused to sit there and listen to her sisters insinuate that she was fat, and they were better than her.

She screamed and swore at them. She called them names. She accused them of being rude, insensitive, and hurtful. She promised she would never, as long as she lived, ever forgive either one of them for triggering her unpleasant and painful thoughts and feelings about herself. She stood up so abruptly and with such force, her chair tumbled over.

Mellie and Louisa both sat dumbfounded as the door slammed, and they heard Darlene screech out of the driveway. "What the hell just happened?" they wondered, and "Is she going to be okay?"

When she got home, she went straight to her computer. She knew her group of online friends would help her feel better. They'd understand her anguish. They would support her.

Before she shared her horrible story, she read about another member who had just confronted her lifelong best friend. She told her, "I don't want to see any more pictures of you. I understand you're happy with your looks, but as someone who is fatter than you and hates her body, you need to understand how pictures of your thin body make me feel even worse about myself. If you're going to continue posting pictures of yourself on your Facebook page, knowing that they are triggering terrible feelings about myself, then I will have to cut you out of my life...forever!"

The comments on her post were all some variation of "Yay! Good for you for taking care of yourself." "You don't need people like her in your life." "Get rid of her." "Way to stand up for yourself."

Darlene was mad. She was mad as hell. She could spit nails. But she wasn't so mad she couldn't pause for a minute. This girl just threatened to end her relationship with her best friend. Sharing Darlene's story would prompt the same suggestions to end her relationship with Mellie and Louisa.

These were her sisters. Regardless of what just happened, she wasn't about to cut them out of her life, not over this. They'd been her best friends since she was born.

She sat for a long time and thought. She saw the absurdity in telling someone you don't want to see any pictures where they look good because it makes you feel bad. That would be like telling someone, "I don't want to see your wedding photos because I want to get married, and I don't have a boyfriend, and seeing you in love triggers me to feel sorry for myself."

Darlene knows how to use the Silver Lining Cycle. She knew she had the power to change how she was feeling. She'd just been in Mean Girl default cycle. She fell back on what she'd always done and looked for others to change so she would feel good about herself. Darlene was in the place that felt most familiar to her. And Mean Girl shared that comfortable space with her, keeping her from venturing into new, unchartered territory where she could take hold of the reigns, grow as a person, and adjust what she thought and felt about what her sisters said.

Darlene felt horrible. She knew it. She felt it in her body. She also recognized she had the power to make it go away. That's exactly what she wanted to do.

Mean Girl believed it's better to be safe than to experience discomfort. If her sisters are willing to cause her pain, she's better off without them. They engage in the following dialog:

Mean Girl praises, "You did the right thing. You should never forgive them for how blatantly they attacked you."

Darlene responds, "These are my sisters. Why would they intentionally gang up on me and make me feel horrible about myself."

Mean Girl declares, "They are both selfish and inconsiderate."

Darlene feels the heat of her anger rise as she considers what Mean Girl said. But she's trying to think this out so she can reduce her anger, not increase it. Relationships are never healed through conflict or battles. The relationship with her sisters won't heal through conflict and neither will her relationship with Mean Girl. Even though Mean Girl addresses Darlene with scorn, she decides not to fight fire with fire and instead neutralize Mean Girl by presenting an opposing opinion. "No. They're not horrible people."

Mean Girl lashes out. "Well then, if they're not horrible, explain why they would do this."

Darlene says, "I know it doesn't make sense. I'll find the answer."

Mean Girl argues, "Yeah, right. You haven't found an answer in your entire life."

Darlene responds, "I've come up with plenty of good answers."

Mean Girl taunts, "Not as good as the ones I've come up with."

Darlene sings a line, "Hush little Mean Girl... Let me think... My sisters both love and care about me. They don't want to hurt me."

Mean Girl calms down a little and questions, "Then why did they?"

Darlene thinks for a moment. "I don't know. Maybe it's not really about me. Maybe they're judging themselves and not judging me."

Mean Girl wonders, "Why would they be judging themselves?"

Darlene says, "Could Mellie be feeling self-conscious in a bathing suit? She is so pretty. She has no reason to feel self-conscious."

Mean Girl reminds, "She hurt your feelings, don't you want to do the same to her?"

Darlene states, "No. I would never intentionally try to hurt Mellie as revenge."

Mean Girl can't argue with that as Darlene would never intentionally hurt someone else's feelings. That's not to say she doesn't do it on accident from time to time, but that's not part of this dialogue.

Darlene wonders, "Why is Louisa taking pills to keep from eating sweets? That's so unhealthy. Maybe I overreacted?"

Sometimes we get hit so fast with a situation, it's difficult to rationally decide the best thing to think, feel, or do. This was one of those situations. At this point, Darlene couldn't do anything about the cycle that caused her to storm out, but she could create a cycle to help her gain control over what just happened.

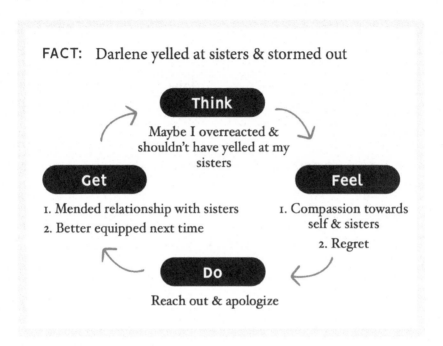

FACT: Darlene yelled at sisters & stormed out

Think
Maybe I overreacted & shouldn't have yelled at my sisters

Feel
1. Compassion towards self & sisters
2. Regret

Do
Reach out & apologize

Get
1. Mended relationship with sisters
2. Better equipped next time

There are a couple of things to notice here. Mean Girl's negative comments and Darlene's compassionate thoughts can't occupy the same space. Think about it for a minute. If you're petting a puppy and it's licking your face and bouncing around, you can't be thinking, "This is the cutest puppy ever, I just love it so much, and its little tongue tickles when it touches my face," and at the same time think, "I'm so fat and worthless, I'll probably never make enough money, and we'll end up losing the house." That's why pets reduce stress. So once Darlene shifted her thoughts to something that evoked compassion toward her sisters, she started to feel more at ease and think more rationally.

We're always going to experience situations where someone says or does something and we feel angry and upset. That's okay. We're not always going to respond or address the situation in a healthy, mature manner. That's okay too. It's not easy, all we can do is try not to react impulsively. When we do, take what we can learn and apply it next time we're in a similar situation. For example, Darlene wasn't in the right space at the time, but with growth, practice, and applying what she learned, next time she might be able to create a cycle that looks like this:

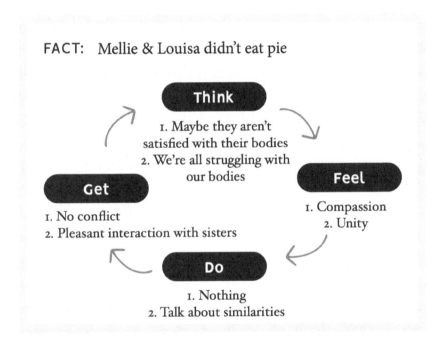

FACT: Mellie & Louisa didn't eat pie

Think
1. Maybe they aren't satisfied with their bodies
2. We're all struggling with our bodies

Feel
1. Compassion
2. Unity

Do
1. Nothing
2. Talk about similarities

Get
1. No conflict
2. Pleasant interaction with sisters

The other thing to notice here is that when Darlene got home and started thinking about the situation, she didn't let Mean Girl call the shots. Instead, they had a conversation with opposing opinions. This strategy can be fun. I used to play the opposite game in the car when my kids were little, and now I play it with my grandbabies. You can play the opposite game with Mean Girl. For example:

Mean Girl: "You're unmotivated."

You: "I'm very motivated."

Mean Girl: "You're going to fail."

You: "I'm going to knock this outta the park."

Mean Girl: "You're fat and ugly."

You: "I'm the most beautiful person in the whole wide world."

This strategy isn't necessarily to convince you that the things you're saying are true, so it's okay if you don't fully believe the opposites you toss back at her. In fact, you can go completely over the top. If she says, "You're broke and don't have any money," you can respond by saying, "I get paid so much, I have more money than the richest person in the world." Mean Girl doesn't have the skill to develop her own language, she just emulates what she hears. This strategy helps broaden her language base so she has other things to say besides just the trash talk she's used to hearing.

Back to these events Darlene refers to as "triggers". They are simply external circumstances that generate unpleasant thoughts in her head. They make her feel anxious and bothered because she hasn't explored them yet. She labels them "triggers" because they make her feel unsettled. We use words to help us make sense of how we feel and how we fit into the world around us. When television and media introduced the word *trigger* to describe things that make us feel agitated, it made perfect sense that Darlene would use that word to describe what she was experiencing.

Mellie didn't trigger any past trauma for Darlene when she said she didn't want any dessert. She simply made a statement, and Darlene attached a bunch of thoughts about herself to that statement that caused her to feel bad. That's really not Mellie's or Louisa's fault.

Darlene was ill at ease and unaccepting of herself. It felt impossible to make herself happy. Like anything else that's overwhelming, she thought it would be much easier if someone did it for her. So, she looked for everyone else to make her happy. Not only is that unrealistic, but it also puts a huge burden on the people around her. Her happiness is a big job; it's one of those things that if she wants it done right, she better do it herself regardless of how difficult it is.

Darlene needed to continue to be a more active participant in her life. Like Darlene, you have the power to choose whether or not you're going to get worked up when someone makes a comment or voices an opposing opinion about food, diet, body size, or weight. You also have the power to choose whether or not you're going to give in to Mean Girl. Like Darlene, you are in charge of your own growth process. Darlene was on the right track as she continued taking responsibility by not letting Mean Girl sit in the driver's seat and choosing not to stay in default mode and falling back on what she's always done in the past.

What happened with Darlene in this chapter is an excellent example of the value of letting go of toxic relationships. In this situation, her relationship with her sisters was not toxic, and she was very clear in her mind she wasn't willing to let it go. However, the online group she participates in may be toxic enough to let go.

Now that Darlene is in a place where she's better equipped to take control of her own happiness, let's turn to the next chapter and see how she starts to mend her relationship with her body.

* * *

MEAN GIRL STRATEGY:

Play the opposite game with Mean Girl. For example:

When Mean Girl says, "You're unmotivated."
You say, "I'm very motivated."

When Mean Girl says, "You're going to fail."
You say, "I'm going to knock this outta the park."

When Mean Girl says, "You're fat and ugly."
You say, "I'm the most beautiful person in the whole wide world."

This strategy isn't necessarily to convince you that the things you're saying are true, so it's okay if you don't fully believe the opposites you toss back at her. In fact, you can go completely over the top. If she says, "You're broke and don't have any money," you can respond by saying, "I get paid so much, I have more money than the richest person in the world." Mean Girl doesn't have the skill to develop her own language, she just emulates what she hears. This strategy helps broaden her language base so she has other things to say besides just the trash talk she's used to hearing.

❧ 9 ❧

MEAN GIRL LIE:

IF MY ASS WERE SMALLER, LIFE WOULD BE PERFECT

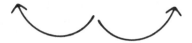

All the hope in the world won't change your predetermined size and shape, which are strongly determined by genetics. No matter how motivated you are. No matter how hard you try. No matter how much willpower you have. You can't change the body size your genes created. Not any more than you can change your height, the length of your fingers, or the width of your feet.

Darlene didn't believe how much genetics determined her body's appearance, so she started going to the gym. Don't get me wrong, our bodies were intended to be in motion, and there's nothing wrong with going to the gym, exercising, or wanting to feel strong. It's a different story when you're trying to chase an impossible dream. Darlene was serious and she meant business. She laid out the cash and hired a personal trainer who asked about her goals. Darlene confessed she wanted her body to look ten years younger than her actual age. Her trainer had her bring in some photos of what she had in mind so she could guide her. Darlene brought in pictures of Jennifer Aniston's arms and shoulders, Britney Spears's belly, and Julia Roberts's legs. They created a plan and Darlene set out to work. She worked hard every day. Her journey toward the body of her dreams had begun. Soon her life would be perfect.

What's bizarre about this is that Darlene's trainer acted like she was creating a custom-designed wedding gown where the bride chooses her favorite sleeves, her favorite bodice, and her favorite skirt. In the end, she'll have a perfect, one-of-a-kind wedding dress. Except Darlene was already a perfect one of a kind. Yet she still believed if she were smaller, her life would be perfect, and with the support, encouragement, and reinforcement from her trainer, she stuck with it.

This is an outrageous example of how the weight loss industry tries to convince people there's something wrong with their bodies then offers to sell them something to fix it. There's a lot of money to be made from people's dissatisfaction with their bodies, and they are willing to sell you an unrealistic result.

As I said, there is nothing wrong with wanting to move your body. There is nothing wrong with wanting to feel strong. But don't let anyone convince you that you can sculpt, contour, lift, or spot reduce specific body parts. Every body is unique and will respond differently. Even if everyone did the same workout, for the same amount of time, and ate the same quantity and type of food, every body would still look different from all the others. As did Darlene's.

It was impossible for Darlene to keep up the pace her trainer had set for her. She eventually ran out of energy and money to maintain the level of dedication required to obtain the Frankenbody her trainer dangled in front of her. Of course, when things didn't turn out the way she hoped, Mean Girl blamed her. Remember, Mean Girl is a copycat. She mimics things she's already heard. In this case, she repeated diet culture's accusations, blaming Darlene for failing, when it should actually be the other way around: diets failed Darlene, and they have failed you too. So Mean Girl said:

"You just have to want it more."
"If you weren't so lazy and you were more motivated."
"You don't have enough willpower."
"You just need to work harder."
"Nothing tastes as good as skinny feels."
"No pain, no gain."
"Keep your eye on the prize."

No matter what Mean Girl said and no matter how much willpower or hard work Darlene put in, she was never going to have Jennifer Aniston's arms and shoulders. Darlene has a different body structure. Julia Roberts reveals in the movie *Pretty Woman*, "My leg is fourty-four inches from hip to toe." Darlene's leg is only thirty-seven inches from hip to toe. It's going to take a lot more than motivation and willpower to extend Darlene's leg seven inches or change the natural structure of her upper body.

What's really unfortunate is Darlene thought her inability to create the body of her dreams was her own damn fault. If this was your friend, what would you think, what would you tell her?

WHAT WILL BE DIFFERENT?

In addition to Darlene's workout routine, she was on a diet that included severe restriction. She ate from a very strict food list and only during a four-hour window. The other twenty hours of the day, no matter how hungry she got, she'd only drink water. She lost weight, yet she was still miserable. Would she ever be small enough? She hoped so. So, she kept trying, but, as with the exercise program, she just couldn't stick with it and finally gave up.

As with most diets, when the restriction ends, your body goes into storage mode. We'll talk more about that later. As summer turned into fall and fall into winter, Darlene's body did just that. As winter drifted toward spring then summer came back around, Darlene was just as unhappy with her size and appearance as she always was. Her weight went up, then it went down, and then back up. The only thing that was consistent during the diet cycle was Darlene never once felt small enough, good enough, or deserving enough.

WHAT IF YOUR BODY CHANGED?

She was so tired and frustrated, she wished she could take a magic pill (which doesn't exist, by the way) and wake up the next day with the body of her dreams. If this pill did exist, besides her size, what would be different from last night when she went to bed? Ask yourself what would be different? Would your closets need to be organized? Would you have neglected leftovers growing in your refrigerator? Would you have the same bills? The same bank balance? The same job? The same income? The same nagging mother-in-law? The same cluttered basement? The same kids who spill milk on the floor? The same husband who leaves the gas tank on empty? Seriously, what is it we think is going to be so dramatically different?

None of these things are going to change with the size of your body. So, besides what you think about your body and what you think other people think about your body, write out on a sheet of paper what would be different? What would you actually do differently if you woke up tomorrow with the body of your dreams? How would you act? How would you present yourself? What would you think? How would your place in the world be different? What would you do differently that's within your control? Look over your list and now ask yourself, what are the thoughts that are keeping you from doing all those things right now with the body you have?

WHAT IF YOUR BODY NEVER CHANGES?

Is it possible to love something that isn't perfect? Or something that isn't exactly what you hoped for, wanted, or expected? Reality doesn't always match your expectations. But still, when it happens, do you immediately jump straight to hate as quickly as you do when it comes to your body?

Maybe it rained on your wedding day, and your outdoor photos have umbrellas instead of sunshine, or your poor dog can't hear then she loses her vision.

Maybe you have physical aches, pains, and injuries, or even chronic limitations that interfere with your quality of life. Your body might not look the way you want it to or the way it used to.

I've never heard anyone say they hated their wedding or their dog. Yet I've heard countless women declare, "I hate my body."

Imagine you're in an unfulfilling relationship with your significant other. You say things like, "I will never love him. I hate everything about him. I can't stand to look at him. He's ugly. I'm ashamed of him. I don't want anyone to see him. I talk bad about him. I treat him poorly. I don't take care of him. I don't do anything to make him feel good. I neglect him. He's an embarrassment."

That sounds like a really stressful and unhealthy relationship. So much animosity could easily spill into other areas of your life, such as your job, other relationships, self-esteem, even your health. Family, friends, your doctor, or anyone else who cares about you would probably suggest and support you in relieving some of the stress related to your relationship with your partner. I'm sure if one of your friends were talking about their marriage this way, you'd be concerned. I know I would be if someone I loved was in a similar situation. What is concerning is that so many women are in relationships just like this, not with other people, but with their own body. Let me repeat the monologue from above except this time replacing "him/he" with "my body." Does this sound familiar?

"I will never love my body. I hate everything about my body. I can't stand to look at my body. My body is ugly. I'm ashamed of my body. I don't want anyone to see my body. I talk bad about my body. I treat my body poorly. I don't take care of my body. I don't do anything to make my body feel good. I neglect my body. My body is an embarrassment."

There's a lot going on here. Let's take a look at the Silver Lining Cycle.

The FACT here is you have a body.

The cycle looks like this:

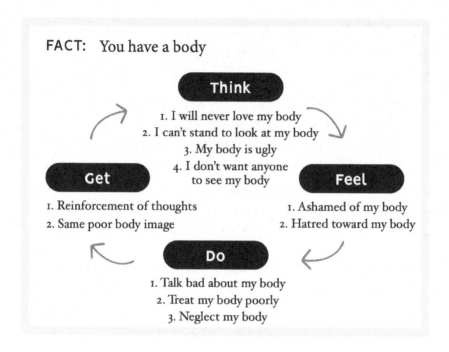

FACT: You have a body

Think

1. I will never love my body
2. I can't stand to look at my body
3. My body is ugly
4. I don't want anyone to see my body

Get

1. Reinforcement of thoughts
2. Same poor body image

Feel

1. Ashamed of my body
2. Hatred toward my body

Do

1. Talk bad about my body
2. Treat my body poorly
3. Neglect my body

The only purpose of this vicious cycle is to keep you stuck and hold you back. It keeps you from growing and moving toward a loving relationship with yourself. It prevents you from becoming the person you want to be. In order to love yourself, you have to accept yourself as a whole. Your body is a part of that whole. You don't have to love your body to love yourself, but you do have to accept it as it is.

WHERE DO WE START?

You have choices. You can change what you think, what you feel, or what you do. Before we get to that, it's important that we acknowledge this is a sensitive topic and a tough chapter. You may have some strong feelings about things not turning out the way you hoped they would. That's okay. Most of us, including me, believed society, the media, and the $72-billion weight loss industry when they told us we should and could achieve a dream body. You're not going through this alone.

You don't have to change the thought to change the cycle. Remember, it's not linear, you can interrupt the cycle by starting at any point. You can change by asking yourself, "How do I want to feel about my body?" While you're the only one who can truly answer that question, I can give some examples of how others have answered.

How do I want to FEEL about my body? Examples include:

- Grateful (it's the only one I have)
- Accepting
- Secure in my appearance

What do I need to DO? Examples include:

- Change your self-talk to things that better serve you
- Treat your body with care and respect
- Do things to make your body feel good (warm bath, massage, etc.)
- Feed it according to its needs

What will you GET? Examples include:

- Improved body image
- Improved self-esteem
- Increased confidence

When I get that what will I THINK? Examples include:

- Media, society, and the weight loss industry lied when they tried to convince me that I needed to change my body in order to feel good.
- My body is not a reflection of who I am as a person.

There's a worksheet on my website to run the Silver Lining Cycle on these questions for yourself—www.julieglynn.com.

Answering each of these questions honestly can be very difficult as they challenge beliefs we've been carrying around for years. But self-compassion is the most effective first step toward improving your relationship with your body.

TURN YOUR COMPASSION FOR OTHERS TOWARD YOURSELF

When Darlene was on a diet, her body hatred was at its highest. Whenever she was preoccupied with food and exercise, she was also hyper-focused on the imperfections of her body. During these periods of dieting, she would turn down invitations to parties and events because she was dieting, believed she didn't have anything to wear, or because she hated how she looked. She made up an excuse not to attend her cousin's wedding because she couldn't find a dress she thought looked good on her. She canceled a cruise with her husband because she refused to wear a bathing suit. She hadn't attended a single class reunion because she hated how she looked and didn't want anyone to see her.

How does it make you feel to hear that Darlene is living like this? Sometimes the best way to cultivate self-compassion is to be in touch with your compassion for others and then turn it toward yourself. Now, think about someone you care about who you think is beautiful. I'm not talking about physical beauty. Think of someone you think is a beautiful soul. What if she declined invitations to events or to hang around you because she hates how she looks? What if she was attending events but secretly suffering because she hated her body? She's ashamed. She's embarrassed. She doesn't want anyone to see her, and she'd rather be at home. Slow down here a minute and really give some deep thought to the question. How would you feel if someone you love and care about hated her body so much she was compromising her quality of life?

Take out a piece of paper and write down all the things you would say to help *her* feel loved and supported. Don't bother with grammar or sentence structure, just dump all your thoughts as they come. What would you tell her? Is there something you want her to know about herself? Do you see something in her that she doesn't see?

Stop and come back when you're done.

How did that feel? As I said, sometimes the best way to cultivate self-compassion is to tap into our compassion for others and then turn it toward ourselves. Now I'm going to invite you to do another activity.

Imagine the person you were just writing to is trying to help you. Take what you just wrote and read it, but instead of reading it to her, picture your friend saying all these things to you. How does it feel hearing that?

Earlier we talked about how Darlene thought her inability to create the body of her dreams was her own damn fault. Do this same exercise and write down the things you would say to a friend who thought it was her fault she never achieved her dream body. Then reread it as if your friend was saying it to you.

DON'T TURN OTHER PEOPLE'S THOUGHTS AGAINST YOU

It's important to notice how much of your body hatred exists inside your head. You look in the mirror then attach a thought to what you see. Remember, mirrors only reflect what you look like on the outside, not who you are on the inside. Then you go out in public and take those thoughts and put them in everyone else's heads—people you don't know, just anyone who happens to walk by. You guess they are thinking the same nasty, unpleasant, and harsh thoughts that usually pop up in your head. The same ones Mean Girl repeats about your body, appearance, food choices, you name it.

It's bad enough dealing with Mean Girl in your own head, let's not also put her in other people's heads to use against you. What other people are thinking is not your responsibility or your problem. Their thoughts are none of your business. You aren't here for other people to look at. You certainly aren't here to be aesthetically pleasing to anyone. Your time and energy are better spent focusing on yourself and your own thoughts.

Truth is, most people are so wrapped up in their own lives, they're probably spending way less time thinking about you than you think. And it's more likely they aren't even thinking about you at all.

I'd like to tell you to simply stop worrying about what other people think. That's a big leap I don't expect you to do overnight, so here's a baby step you can take until you're no longer guessing what people are thinking about you. It's important to follow the Silver Lining Cycle and make sure if you're going to guess, you're at least choosing thoughts that make you feel good instead of things that make you feel unworthy.

When you walk past someone, instead of thinking, "They just noticed my neck fat," choose to think, "They have no idea how friendly and funny I am."

It's not that easy to grab a feel-good thought in an instant, so it may be a good idea to have a list on standby ready and waiting for these types of situations. Take out another sheet of paper and make a list of positive things about yourself. If you can't think of anything, ask your friends. Tell them, "I'm creating a list of my positive traits; can you think of anything I should put on the list?"

OKAY, SO LET'S SAY I ACCEPT MY BODY. WHAT ABOUT MY HEALTH?

While appearance doesn't equal worth, weight doesn't necessarily equal health. I think it is fascinating that many of the chronic health factors associated with weight are also the same as those associated with stress. For example, heart disease, high blood pressure, headaches, and breathing problems are overlapping health factors for both stress and weight.

It's disturbing that when it comes to our health, consideration is rarely given to the amount of stress people might experience when they have a toxic relationship with their own bodies. Perhaps stress levels resulting from hating and trying to reshape your body should be addressed before adding more stress to the body through dieting and creating an internal fear of starvation.

Every time Darlene went to the doctor, he asked about external stressors she might be experiencing (relationships, job, family, etc.) Unfortunately, Darlene's medical team has never asked about the stress she might be experiencing based on the relationship she has with herself and her body. On more than one occasion, even with vital signs within the normal range, Darlene's been told to go home and create additional stress on her body by putting it into starvation mode (aka dieting) and exercising more.

If you know your stress is increased as a result of the relationship you have with your body, I congratulate you on reading this book, and I encourage you to do the suggested activities that will help alleviate some of the stress.

WHAT ABOUT MEAN GIRL?

Mean Girl is probably more vocal and critical when it comes to bodies than she is about anything else. This is one of my favorite strategies to help her calm down. (That's not really true. All the strategies are my favorite, but this one is kind of fun.)

Once a day, take a sheet of paper and write down all the judgmental thoughts Mean Girl says about your body. If you want, you can include other things too. Every judgment and every negative statement, every criticism she makes. Writing them down gets all the negative thoughts out of your head. It's like clearing the lint filter of your dryer. Clean out the unnecessary blockage so you can have better airflow (thought flow). When you've completed your list, take the sheet of paper and rip it into as many pieces as you can and throw them into the trash. Anything that was listed on that sheet of paper is off-limits for Mean Girl for the rest of the day.

Rather than just crumpling it up and tossing it out, I believe there's a greater level of satisfaction in tearing it and ripping it and shredding it into pieces. And then to add even more satisfaction, I add one more thing to this strategy.

There's a line from the movie *My Cousin Vinny* I think about every time I'm ripping up my paper. If you haven't seen the movie, Vinny is an inexperienced attorney from New York City who took the bar exam six times before he finally passed. For his first case, he's defending his wrongly accused cousin on charges of murdering a 'good old boy' in small-town Alabama. At the start of the trial, the prosecuting attorney presents the jury with an extensive opening statement. Vinny's opening statement to the jury is short and simple. He gets up, walks over to the jury, points to the prosecutor and simply says, "Everything that guy just said is bullshit. Thank you." Then he sits down.

That's what I say as I'm ripping up my paper. "Everything that girl just said is bullshit."

Let's go on to the next chapter and see how Mean Girl affects Darlene's career.

* * *

ACTIVITY:

Besides what you think about your body and what you think other people think about your body, write out on a sheet of paper what would be different? What would you actually do differently if you woke up tomorrow with the body of your dreams? How would you act? How would you present your-self? What would you think? How would your place in the world be different? What would you do differently that's within your control? Look over your list and now ask yourself, what are the thoughts that are keeping you from doing all those things right now with the body you have?

Think about someone you care about who you think is beau-tiful. I'm not just talking about physical beauty. Think of someone you think is beautiful both inside and out. What if she declined invitations to events or to hang around you because she hates how she looks? What if she was attending events but secretly suffering because she hated her body? She's ashamed. She's embarrassed. She doesn't want anyone to see her, and she'd rather be at home. Slow down here a minute and really give some deep thought to the question. How would you feel if someone you love and care about hated her body so much, she was compromising her quality of life?

Take out a piece of paper and write down all the things you would say to help her feel loved and supported. Don't bother with grammar or sentence structure, just dump all your thoughts as they come. What would you tell her? Is there something you want her to know about herself? Do you see something in her that she doesn't see?

Stop and come back when you're done.

Now imagine the person you were just writing to is trying to help you. Take what you just wrote and read it, but instead of reading it to her, picture your friend saying all these things to you. How does it feel hearing that?

Earlier we talked about how Darlene blamed herself for her inability to create the body of her dreams through diet and exercise. Do this same exercise and write down the things you would say to a friend who thought it was her fault she never achieved her dream body. Then reread it as if your friend were saying it to you.

Take out another sheet of paper and make a list of positive things about yourself. If you can't think of anything, ask your friends. Tell them, "I'm creating a list of my positive traits; can you think of anything I should put on the list?" Use this list as a go-to when you're trying to guess what other people are thinking about you instead of giving them a thought that makes you feel bad about yourself.

MEAN GIRL STRATEGY:

Once a day, take a sheet of paper and write down all the judgmental thoughts Mean Girl says about your body. If you want, you can include other things too. Every judgment and every negative statement, every criticism she makes. Writing them down gets all the negative thoughts out of your head. It's like clearing the lint filter of your dryer. Clean out the unnecessary blockage so you can have better airflow (thought flow). When you've completed your list, take the sheet of paper and rip it into as many pieces as you can and throw them into the trash. Anything that was listed on that sheet of paper is off-limits for Mean Girl for the rest of the day.

❧ 10 ❧

MEAN GIRL LIE:

I'M NOT SMART ENOUGH. I'LL FAIL

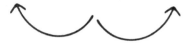

Darlene always loved property. She loved going to open houses. She loved HGTV. She loved tearing down walls, painting, and remodeling. It seemed so natural to incorporate her hobby into a career. So, she became a realtor. Logistically and emotionally, Darlene thought it was a brilliant idea. Mean Girl had a different idea. She did everything she could to persuade Darlene to give it up before she even started.

She heckled, "What makes you think you can sell a house? You probably couldn't sell lemonade in front of a house."

Darlene believed Mean Girl when she insisted, "You don't have what it takes. Nobody will take you seriously. Everyone knows you're a fraud."

Darlene completely agreed when Mean Girl attacked her appearance, "You're not at all presentable or put together. Your clothes are too tight and unprofessional. You're a complete wreck."

And Darlene couldn't argue when Mean Girl accused "You're way too old and uneducated. You'll make a damn fool of yourself. Just stay home, watch HGTV, and save yourself the embarrassment."

Darlene was deflated. She knew Mean Girl was right, so she didn't put any effort into building her real estate career. She got her license then some business cards but didn't do much beyond that. On very rare occasions, she might hand a card out or admit she was a realtor, but only if someone flat out asked her, "What do you do for work?"

Darlene didn't have any confidence. She rarely went into her home office, and when she did, she just sat and watched the neighbor out the window. Sometimes she read books or attended online webinars or participated in realtor groups. She didn't know why she bothered; whenever she read a post about someone's success, she immediately dismissed it. She thought they were luckier or smarter than her. It was so unfair.

Darlene tried to think of ways to get clients, yet she never implemented any of her ideas. She didn't go to networking events or put out ads. She didn't tell her friends she was a realtor. She simply sat around and waited and hoped something would happen. When it didn't, it left her feeling even more like a failure.

So what was going on? Was Darlene too fat to sell real estate? No.

Was Darlene too incompetent to sell real estate? No.

Did Darlene need to be more likable to sell real estate? No.

Did Darlene need to be thinner or prettier to sell real estate? No.

Was Darlene too old to sell real estate? No.

So why couldn't Darlene sell real estate?

Darlene couldn't sell real estate because she didn't think she could. She was scared and lacked confidence. She was afraid of failing, so she refused to even try. She felt she was better off not trying at all than trying and failing. At least that way she had an excuse when things didn't work out.

The fact is realtors come in all shapes and sizes. Darlene was smart enough to pass the realtor exam; she was certainly smart enough to sell real estate. There wasn't any concrete evidence to support Darlene's fear that she would fail as a realtor other than her own thoughts. The problem is, Darlene was immobilized by Mean Girl controlling her negative thinking.

Darlene needed to take control. The first strategy she implemented was either pairing Mean Girl's statements with a positive *and* or by preceding them with *even though* followed by a positive statement.

When Mean Girl heckled, "You are going to screw this up."

Darlene responded, "Even though I might screw this up, I can still try."

When Mean Girl insisted, "Nobody will take you seriously."

Darlene said, "Even though people might not take me seriously, I have the skills to sell real estate."

When Mean Girl attacked her appearance, "Your clothes are too tight and unprofessional."

Darlene countered, "And I can still negotiate on behalf of a client."

When Mean Girl accused, "You're way too old and uneducated."

Darlene rebutted, "And I am younger than many other people who also have passed the same exam I did."

Of course, Darlene doesn't completely believe her responses. That's okay. That's not the point of this strategy. The goal is to give Mean Girl new ideas and tools to use to support you. It's like filling a bucket of sand one teaspoon at a time. It's going take a while, but every teaspoon you drop in the bucket fills it just a little bit more. Each follow-up comment is like one little teaspoon filling Mean Girl with new ideas.

You can make this fun and outlandish if you want. When Mean Girl says, "You're a complete wreck." You can respond,

"I'm a complete wreck, and I'm too sexy for my shirt; so sexy it hurts, so I do a little turn on the catwalk."

Another strategy she used was reframing Mean Girl with more realistic thoughts. She asked Mean Girl, "What's the worst thing that could realistically happen if I put myself out there?"

Only Darlene really knows the answer to that question. If I had to guess, I'd say the worst thing is nothing changes, and Darlene never gets any clients and never sells a house. Since Darlene already agreed to stop putting Mean Girl's thoughts into other people's heads to use against her and she's also accepted it's her own thoughts that create her feelings, she can't use what other people might think or say as one of the worst things that could happen.

Growth is very scary for Mean Girl. So, if the worst thing that could realistically happen is things stay exactly the same, she really has nothing to fear.

As I've said, I believe we can elicit change at any spot on the Silver Lining Cycle. In this situation, Darlene's thoughts and feelings have imprisoned her with inactivity. Her best option was to change her thoughts.

This is an example of the negative cycle Darlene was trapped in:

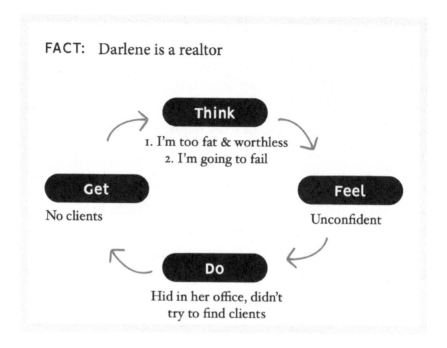

FACT: Darlene is a realtor

Think
1. I'm too fat & worthless
2. I'm going to fail

Feel
Unconfident

Do
Hid in her office, didn't
try to find clients

Get
No clients

Here's a better option, a positive cycle, that's available once
Darlene addressed Mean Girl and shifted her thoughts:

FACT: Darlene is a realtor

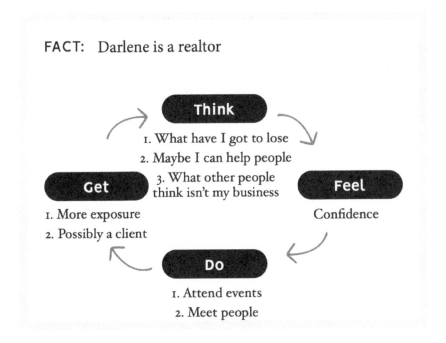

Changing that thought to "What have I got to lose?" or "I can help people" will make a difference. Remembering that what other people think about her isn't her business gave Darlene the confidence she needed to make a small change. Again, it's important to mention, Darlene didn't commit to meeting a thousand people a day and getting two hundred clients in a week. She took it one small step at a time. She committed to attending one event. What was really beneficial for her is that one action step reinforced her new thoughts and created more confidence, so she was able to commit to taking one more small step.

Years ago, I was a Mary Kay Consultant. I remember being at one of those meetings where they try to get people to sign up to sell the product. Someone in the audience asked the question, "What percentage of Mary Kay ladies actually get a pink Cadillac?" The answer was amazing, "100% of the women who don't give up until they've gotten one." There was no reason Darlene couldn't be one of those women who didn't give up until she reached her goal. All she had to do was be aware of Mean Girl. She had to remember Mean Girl's job was to keep her safe. Then she had to respond to Mean Girl and her circumstances with different thoughts and strategies.

When Mean Girl said, "You'll screw this up and embarrass yourself."

Darlene acknowledged that Mean Girl means well, and she responds, "That's okay. I've screwed things up and embarrassed myself before, and that doesn't mean I'm going to screw this up too."

Embarrassment is caused by our thoughts, especially when we think we should have responded or acted differently than we did. Once I accidentally ordered a package of happy birthday cookies and had them sent to my friend when her dad died. She thanked me for the birthday cookies and the note about her father. I had no idea what she was talking about. She told me she thought I did it on purpose to make her laugh. I didn't. Then she laughed even harder when she found out I somehow managed to totally screw up my cookie order. It shouldn't be that hard, right? I mean, who messes up and accidentally sends happy birthday cookies when they meant to send sympathy cookies? I did and I was okay with it. So was my friend. So was Mean Girl. I screw things up sometimes, and that doesn't mean I'm going to screw everything up.

Mean Girl says, "You're not thin enough or pretty enough to sell real estate."

Darlene says, "Even though I'm not thin, I can still sell real estate."

If Darlene believed Mean Girl when she told her she needed to change her size, shape, or appearance as a prerequisite for taking action, she would always be at a standstill. As we all know, we can spend a lifetime trying to change how we look and never achieve long-term satisfaction. Changing her size isn't going to change her ability to succeed. Changing her thoughts will.

Mean Girl says, "You're too weak and lazy."

Darlene says, "And yet, I still learn and grow."

Darlene sometimes saw herself as weak, lazy, and unmotivated. We all do from time to time; that doesn't mean we don't still learn and grow. The lifetime Darlene spent obsessing about weight, dieting, food, cooking, and exercise took a ton of learning, energy, dedication, focus, and strength.

She counted calories. She memorized point values. She learned everything there was to know about macros. She interpreted a Ketostix. She learned how to cook. She planned meals. Then she modified recipes using coconut instead of flour, zucchini instead of pasta. Her favorites were cauliflower instead of potatoes, instead of pizza crust, instead of rice, instead of macaroni, instead of breadsticks, instead of grilled cheese, instead of bagels, instead of nachos, and instead of Reece's Peanut Butter Cups. Okay, she never mastered that last one, but I thought I'd throw it in for fun.

She sourced hard-to-find ingredients. She measured and weighed both her food and her body. She documented points, portions, fats, proteins, liquids, exercise, distances, times, weights, and measurements.

She read labels. She read books. She asked questions. She attended meetings and started online groups. She created a cookbook. She set the clock and followed strict feeding times. She created little tricks to fool her body into thinking she was full when she was starving.

How could we accuse someone with that much devotion of being weak, lazy, or unmotivated? Imagine what she will accomplish now that she's shifted all that time and mental energy away from dieting and weight loss and focused it instead on her new career.

Darlene isn't alone. Countless women have spent as many years and as much time as she has dominated by the promises of the $72-billion weight loss industry. Here are some of the things women have told me they've accomplished since they let go of diets and the weight loss mentality. After all, nourishing your body shouldn't be a lifelong full-time job.

- I literally started a business. I have FINALLY had the mental capacity to make it an official business. I opened a bank account, and today I created a website.
- I discovered jewelry making.
- I am experimenting with essential oils.
- I'm able to read and rest my mind, whereas calorie

counting had me constantly researching foods and breaking down macros. It was such a pain.

- I'm writing a blog.
- I've been traveling. I went to Myanmar and Malaysia, and I'm learning to speak Myanmar (Burmese).
- I started painting again.
- I'm quilting like crazy.
- I decided to go back to graduate school.
- My house is decluttered, organized, and spotless.
- I am teaching myself how to play the piano.
- I'm reading more for pleasure.
- I found a spiritual practice! I discovered I have lots of intuitive abilities, and I am now a practicing psychic medium. All in nine months.
- I'm finally taking my career as a self-published author seriously and putting in the necessary work and focus it takes to build it as a career and not just a hobby.
- I'm spending more relaxed time with my teenage children.

Darlene's story and the accomplishments these women share are excellent examples of how to use the Silver Lining Cycle to change your life. Once these women neutralized food and normalized eating, their thoughts and feelings changed, and so did their actions. In essence, they jumped off the diet hamster wheel and started accomplishing things in their lives.

Take out a sheet of paper and answer these questions:

- What could you accomplish if you shifted your focus

to other things besides diet, weight loss, and body
image?
- Where have you shown strength that you're not
giving yourself credit for?
- Where have you put in the effort and succeeded?
Maybe it was overcoming a difficult situation or
accomplishing a goal.
- Where are you letting fear hold you back?

Okay, so now that you've gotten to a place where you're more
accepting of yourself, and you've got a better relationship
with Mean Girl, let's go on to the next chapter and talk about
feeding the body you've been gifted.

* * *

ACTIVITY:

Take out a sheet of paper and answer these questions:

- What could you accomplish if you shifted your focus
to other things besides diet, weight loss, and body
image?
- Where have you shown strength that you're not
giving yourself credit for?
- Where have you put in the effort and succeeded?
Maybe it was overcoming a difficult situation or
accomplishing a goal.
- Where are you letting fear hold you back?

MEAN GIRL STRATEGY:

Pair Mean Girl's statements with a positive *and*. For example, "They're never going to hire you *and* I'm qualified, so I'm going to apply."

Precede Mean Girl's statement with *even though* and follow it with a positive statement. For example, "*Even though* I have a short attention span, *I can still get things done.*"

Reframe Mean Girl's thoughts with more realistic things. For example, Mean Girl says, "You're going to lose everything you own, including your house, your car, your clothes, your job, and all the people who love you. You'll be all alone on the street looking for a box to curl up in." (Which, by the way, is exactly how Mean Girl wanted to answer the question above about what's the worst thing that could happen if Darlene put effort into her real estate career. Darlene tossed that answer out as way too unrealistic, which is why the example is being used here instead of up there.) Instead, Darlene's reframe was, "Things may never get any better, and worst-case scenario, they will stay exactly the same."

Prepare yourself to rebut some of Mean Girl's comments by practicing these strategies.

Pairing with *and*:

"_____" and "_____"

(Mean Girl says) (You say)

Precede with *even though* and follow it with a positive statement: "Even though _____ , I _____."
(Mean Girl says) (You say)

MEAN GIRL LIE:

I DON'T HAVE ENOUGH MOTIVATION OR WILLPOWER

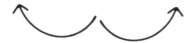

When Darlene was in seventh grade, she and her friends used to ingest over-the-counter appetite suppressant pills in the form of a liquid drop. Why liquid? They hadn't matured enough to successfully swallow a pill without choking. Sometimes out of desperation, when they didn't have a drink to mix it with, they'd just drop them directly into their mouths. Concerning behavior for young, growing junior high school girls.

Darlene has dieted off and on ever since. She tried every weight loss trick she'd ever heard of. Some more than once.

Some more conventional. Some more outlandish. It didn't matter. If there was any chance she'd lose weight, she tried it.

There were times she lost enough weight people noticed and commented. It was never enough. Darlene was never happy with her weight. Never in her entire life had she looked in the mirror or stood on the scale and thought, "Gee, I'm okay with my weight."

She always wanted to lose more and more until she felt so tortured and overworked, her tired and exhausted body just gave up.

Whenever this happened, Mean Girl immediately chastised and berated her.

"All you had to do was try harder."

"You're disgusting."

"You're weak, gross, useless, and lazy."

No matter how much weight Darlene lost, she inevitably gained it all back and sometimes even more.

She didn't understand. Why was she such a huge failure? How could she expect to be successful anywhere else in her life when she continually failed every single diet since she was twelve?

Darlene was so ashamed and embarrassed. The truth is it was no more Darlene's fault she couldn't maintain weight loss from dieting than it was my fault we had a fire.

WHY WASN'T IT HER FAULT?

Weight loss is a $72-billion industry created by people who discovered they could make a lot of money convincing women their bodies are inadequate, then sell them a solution that doesn't work. We've become dependent on their one plan that fits all rules and restrictions, like guardrails to keep us confined inside the lane of diet culture. We've lost all trust in our body's natural ability to guide us. What's super concerning is girls like Darlene, at twelve years old or even younger, already believe their bodies are inadequate.

WHY DON'T DIETS WORK?

Your body's job is to keep you alive. To do that, it works hard to maintain balance. It's called homeostasis. I don't want to get too sciency. But one example of how it works is this: you have a temperature range your body adjusts and keeps balanced. When you get too hot, you sweat, and if you get too cold, you shiver. What some people may not know is your body also has a weight range. Again, without getting all sciency, your individual weight range is determined the same way genetics determines your height, shape of your head, or size of your feet. Just like you can't change any of those, you also can't change your natural weight range.

Somewhere we got this idea, or we were fed this idea from the weight loss industry and the marketers of diet products, that with enough effort and willpower, we can change our natural weight range. When you attempt to change your weight outside your natural range, just like your temperature, your body tries to bring your weight back within your normal range by either adjusting your metabolism or by increasing or decreasing your hunger. That's one of the reasons we gain weight after we stop dieting. Our body is trying to do its job by bringing everything back into balance.

Sometimes after repeated dieting, we screw up our natural range. That's because our body doesn't know the difference between a diet and starvation. For example, let's say you're vacationing in Hawaii and take a fateful trip from a tropic port aboard a tiny ship. Along with six other people, you set out on a three-hour tour. But then the weather starts getting rough, and the tiny ship gets tossed and sets ground on the shores of an uncharted desert isle. There are no phones, no food. It's as primitive as can be. You're hungry, and what little food is available is shared between everyone. You're running a pretty significant calorie deficit. Is this a diet or are you starving? Your body has no idea.

If you're ever rescued and start eating more regularly, just like when you go off a diet, your body will store additional energy in case there's ever another famine. Because it doesn't know the difference between diet and famine, every time you go on a diet, it thinks you're on the brink of starvation. The more your body experiences starvation, the more storage it needs, increasing your weight range. So, our attempts to decrease our weight range actually end up increasing it.

Some bodies, like Darlene's, have experienced regular famines for so many years, it's constantly storing energy whenever possible. So let's say you keep going on these three-hour boat tours. I mean, most people would probably never go again after they ended up stranded, but for the sake of this story, let's say you continually take these boat trips year after year. Each time you wind up shipwrecked on a deserted island. Before too long, you're probably going to start bringing along extra supplies to take with you in expectation of shipwreck. Every time you diet, it's like going on this boat trip; your body is making sure you have enough supplies by storing extra energy for the next bout of inadequate nourishment, we call a diet. This is good news and bad news. The bad news: no matter what you do after you stop dieting (end a famine), your body will probably store energy, and you'll gain weight. The good news: you can put an end to this cycle. How?

STOP DIETING, STOP CREATING SCARCITY

Diets are based on deprivation. When we fear there's an insufficient supply to meet our needs, we tend to respond with an insatiable desire and stockpile or hoard.

Here's an example. Years ago, Darlene lived in an apartment where the electricity went out all the time. The first time it happened, she was totally unprepared. Just like the castaways were unprepared on that first three-hour tour. She didn't have a flashlight or candles or anything to create light. She sat in the dark and freaked out. The second time it happened, she was only slightly more prepared. But the more it happened, and the more she went without power, the more prepared she became. She bought used candles and candlesticks at yard sales and thrift stores. She shopped clearance sales after the holidays and bought all the candles. Anytime the power went out and she had to tap into her stash, the stronger her desire for more candles became. She was afraid she'd never have enough. Darlene no longer lives in that apartment. Other than a rare storm or an even more rare oversight in paying her electric bill, she hasn't experienced a power outage since. Today she doesn't have any more candles than the average person would for the sake of decoration, occasional ambiance, or fragrance.

Let's say you go on one of those boat tours with plenty of supplies and find calm waters and smooth sailing. Three hours later, you're back at the dock. The next trip and the next are exactly the same. Before you know it, those mishaps that ended in shipwreck are distant memories. You're starting to feel confident you no longer need to bring along as many supplies. Just like Darlene and her candles, when you stop dieting and your body stops expecting a famine, it will likely relax and settle into your predetermined weight range.

HOW DO YOU DO THAT?

Feed your body. To do this, Darlene relearned Intuitive Eating. The reason I say she relearned Intuitive Eating instead of just learning is that we're all born intuitive eaters, yet somehow as we get older, we unlearn it and stop eating intuitively. Imagine a hungry baby. It doesn't matter how much they ate that day or if they just ate two hours ago, when they are hungry, they cry for food. They eat until they are full, and then they stop. Have you ever tried to feed a baby that's not hungry? It's nearly impossible. Basically, that's Intuitive Eating. Sure, it sounds simple, and it is. It's just not that easy. Intuitive eating requires a shift in our thinking that goes against years and years of programming. We're always looking for rules and restrictions and tempted by those promises of "guaranteed weight loss or your money back."

Before we go any further, I want to take a little sidestep here. As we grow through this process, it's important to make a clear distinction. Mean Girl and our intuition are not the same thing. Mean Girl has a strong presence. She's loud, mouthy, and demanding. Our intuition, on the other hand, is very subtle and quiet as it gently pulls or draws us in one direction without much thought.

Let's say you set a date to meet a friend for lunch at a local restaurant. As you start to write it in your calendar, the simple idea *I can walk there* passes through your head like a soft breeze on a still day. You block off thirty extra minutes in your calendar for walking time. On the flip side, say you get the idea *Oh I can walk there*, and that's followed with thoughts like:

"If I walk, I won't have to find a parking spot."

"Oh, but it's mostly all uphill."

"But I'll save $8 in parking fees."

"I could listen to my music on the walk."

"It's so hot though, I'll be sweaty when I get there."

That is not your intuition. That's your brain analyzing the pros and cons.

WHAT IS INTUITIVE EATING?

Intuitive Eating involves making peace with food by eating what you want, when you want, and as much as you want, without restriction. Darlene thought that was too good to be true. But, when she thought about it, wasn't that pretty much what she did anytime she wasn't on a diet? How could that be considered Intuitive Eating?

This is where we have to change our thinking. Every time Darlene ended a diet, she just ate, that was it. She didn't pay attention to her body or how it felt. She didn't pay attention to what she felt like eating or how the food tasted. She didn't let her intuition guide her.

As I said, it's simple, but it's not that easy to pay attention to the messages our body sends, particularly when we don't really like our body, and we're not accustomed to listening, much less responding to its guidance.

TEND TO YOUR UNIQUE NEEDS, LIKE A GARDENER

Darlene wanted to start a vegetable garden. Unfamiliar with gardening, she went to the internet for guidance. She found some simple but eye-opening tips. The first suggestion she read was no matter how much care and attention you give your plants, they won't thrive if you don't know their specific needs. For example, some plants do okay with partial sunlight/partial shade, while others require direct sunlight.

Another suggestion said only water plants as often as needed. Some plants need regular watering and moisture. Others require drier conditions with very little water. Darlene learned she needed to check her plants regularly to see how they were doing and make adjustments as needed.

This was beyond belief. Darlene discovered she wasn't following these same suggestions when it came to her own body. She was ignoring her own specific needs by not checking in on her body regularly. She hadn't been evaluating whether or not she was hungry or full. She wasn't noticing if she was even enjoying her food or how she felt after she ate it. She certainly wasn't making any necessary adjustments she might need. Dang. She was taking better care of her plants' needs than she was her own body.

Believe me, it's worth increasing our awareness, opening ourselves up to listening, and then deciding what we want to do about it. For example, when Darlene eats extra cheese garlic nachos with jalapeños at 10:00 p.m. and wakes at 3:00 a.m. with burning in her throat from acid reflux, that's a message from her body. She decides what she wants to do with that message.

I know this is hard. I've been there and I'm going through this too. Sometimes I just want to throw in the towel and have someone give me a set of rules that will guarantee fast weight loss. Because let's face it, the rules have made it really hard to listen and pay attention to what the acid reflux represents, or worse yet, pushing away a half-full plate of really delicious food when our body says it's too full to swallow another bite.

DECIDING WHAT TO EAT?

How often have you been in a situation where someone asks, "What do you feel like having for lunch?" or "What do you feel like having for dinner?" We usually don't give it much thought, and as women, we're so quick to put our needs and wants aside for others, we often answer with the question, "What do you feel like having?" Then we go with whatever they suggested. Seriously. Ask yourself, "What do you feel like having?" Do you feel like having something cold or hot? Soft or crunchy? Hearty or light? This is your life, your body. What do you want to eat? It's not unusual when my husband and I are on long road trips we go through two different drive-throughs for lunch. What's wrong with that? He wants tacos and I want a burger. After you've chosen what you want to eat, make sure you notice whether or not it was satisfying. How did you feel while you were eating it, and how did you feel afterward?

HOW DO WE DO THAT?

You run experiments. What? More science? Think of it more like gathering evidence. You know, like solving a mystery.

What kind of evidence do you gather? Did you like the taste? Did you eat too much, just right, or not enough? How did you feel after you ate? Things like headaches, tummy troubles, tiredness, aches, pains, indigestion, and acid reflux are all messages from your body or little pieces of evidence worth gathering. Do you notice any patterns? Is there any correlation between these messages and something you ate? Or how much you ate? Or what time you ate?

Darlene discovered from her experiments that she doesn't like how it feels to eat beyond full. When she eats too much pizza for dinner, she gets indigestion and can't sleep. Her favorite cookies don't really taste as good as she thought. The bread at her favorite restaurant gives her a headache. She'll have diarrhea within an hour if she eats too many pancakes. A diet Coke at lunch keeps her awake half the night.

It comes naturally to notice things that cause discomfort. We have to pay extra attention to notice any positive changes. The more water Darlene drinks, the more she wants. She feels more energized on the days she drinks a smoothie for breakfast than when she eats cereal or toast. She notices some subtle health benefits from drinking kombucha.

Just like it's important to develop an awareness of Mean Girl, paying attention to your body and how it reacts to certain foods is another area that requires awareness. Once you become aware, it doesn't mean you have to avoid certain foods or intentionally eat others. Just use this new information when making choices.

One night, Darlene went so far as dialing the phone to call her favorite pizzeria when she stopped, thought for a minute, then decided she didn't want to be up all night with indigestion. She put the phone down and made a different choice. That doesn't mean she never eats pizza. Sometimes she goes ahead and makes the call knowing she's going to have indigestion later. Sometimes she eats it a little earlier as that seems to sit better in her stomach.

Keep in mind, you are the expert of your body. Once you start making discoveries, you may find you have some overlapping similarities with other people. The messages from your body, the discoveries, and the decisions you make for yourself are very unique and personal to you and your individual body. Feedback and opinions from others about what works for them is great for them, but doesn't necessarily apply to you. That's okay.

EATING WITH MEAN GIRL

I mentioned earlier how difficult Intuitive Eating can be with Mean Girl in our head. Let's face it, she doesn't like change. Disrupting the familiar and comfortable patterns of diets, rules, and restrictions are the types of changes she sees as a threat to our safety and security. She's going to fight against it. Food is simply nourishment for your body, but Mean Girl will argue some foods are "good," while other foods are "bad." We've been programmed to believe that for so long that Mean Girl will dissuade us from challenging that belief.

Food is neutral. It's just food. Mean Girl learned a long time ago that food is something we earn or something we sacrifice. She's not going to come around too quickly and accept the idea that we don't need punishment or deprivation from future meals because of the food we ate previously. She's going to encourage you to continue using food as a currency or a trade-off. She might suggest, "You had a donut for breakfast, so you can just have one or two plain celery stalks for lunch."

Don't get me wrong. If you love plain celery, and you're excited as hell to eat them for lunch, by all means, go for it. But if you are hungry and want a sandwich and refuse to eat one because you had a donut for breakfast, that's not eating intuitively. Remember, our intuition gently guides us in the right direction. It doesn't bargain, negotiate, or make lists of the pros and cons.

Mean Girl is going to need some retraining. Take notice and be aware when you're trying to listen and follow the quiet voice of your intuition and Mean Girl is shouting in your head. If you're ready to start challenging her, firmly tell her to "STOP," just like we would if our little dog we love so much was barking a warning.

Tell her it's different now and repeat those things we just talked about.

"Food is nourishment."

"Food is neutral."

"Food is not good, bad, or currency. It's just food."

This is a lot of information for one chapter. To summarize, the best way to end the cycle of losing and gaining weight is to stop dieting. Develop an awareness of what your body needs and wants by paying attention to its subtle messages. Use the information you gather when making meal choices. Continue to develop an awareness of Mean Girl.

I'm sure you're thinking, "This sounds possible, but what about emotional eating?" I wouldn't leave that out. In fact, let's go to the next chapter and talk about it.

* * *

MEAN GIRL STRATEGY:

When Mean Girl starts to freak out, firmly tell her to "STOP," just like you would if your little dog you love so much was barking a warning.

Reassure her with new information. Again, this information is just to help broaden her resources so she can be more supportive in the future.

❧ 12 ❧

MEAN GIRL LIE:

I CAN'T BE TRUSTED AROUND FOOD

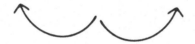

I wrote this chapter three times. The first draft I scrapped. I read through the second draft and considered walking away for a few days. Before I did that, I scrolled back up here to the top and thought maybe I'd go for round three. Here's where the struggle comes in: "emotional eating" stirs up a lot of conflicting thoughts and feelings, as well as all sorts of suggestions about what we should do about it. Most of these imply emotional eating is negative and the result—the GET —is shameful and negative. Here are a few things I found from a quick Google search: "How do I stop emotional eating?" and "How do I gain control over emotional eating?"

There were explanations for why it happens and strategies to help you eliminate emotional eating.

The one that confused me was the question, are you "tired of emotional eating?" Why would anyone be tired of or want to eliminate emotional eating? I guess if we think it's a bad thing, then we'd want to avoid it. The term emotional eating as a stand-alone is simply a statement, it's neutral. It's what we think about emotional eating that makes it bad. If we gave up all emotional eating, what would happen to pleasure eating, celebratory eating, and social eating? There's good and bad in everything. Giving something up completely means we have to give up the good too.

I'm not talking about excessive emotional eating at the root of clinically diagnosed binge eating disorders. This book doesn't cover that topic and isn't intended for anyone currently diagnosed with an active eating disorder or anyone in a program of recovery from addiction. But if you are working to improve your life by changing your thought patterns, keep reading.

In the last chapter, we talked about Intuitive Eating. I mentioned above how emotional eating has been given such a bad reputation. I wonder, can we honestly say with any real certainty that emotional eating is in no way intuitive? Remember, your intuition is natural and very subtle as it gently pulls or draws you in one direction. So, you decide if emotional eating can also be intuitive in any of these scenarios:

- We use food for rewards, celebrations, comfort, and entertainment.
- We connect with people over food.
- Even babies, natural intuitive eaters, bond with their mothers during nursing or are cuddled by those who provide a bottle. Some continue to suckle beyond fullness for comfort.
- Relationships are established, strengthened, and maintained during mealtimes.
- Food has religious and cultural significance.
- Cooking, preparing, presenting, serving, and sharing food is an art form and a gesture of love.
- Providing food for those in need, spiritually, emotionally, or financially is a sign of care and compassion.
- Food is a symbol of love and security. Isn't that why we have sayings like "made with love," "Cooking is love made visible," or "The heart of the home is the kitchen."

All these things seem so natural and essential to human connection and emotional security.

EXAMPLES OF POSITIVE EMOTIONAL EATING

Let's say you're at a wedding. Now, I can't speak for everyone, but I'd guess after enjoying hors d'oeuvres at the cocktail hour and then a fabulously delicious dinner, by the time the couple cuts their cake, very few guests are actually hungry. Yet many guests, myself included, will still eat a piece of wedding cake. We're not eating because we're hungry. We're eating cake to join in the celebration of the happy couple. Some people might even have a second piece, again not because they are hungry, and maybe this slice of cake isn't to celebrate the couple. It might be so damn good and since they'll never get it again, they want a little bit more. That's okay. There's no reason to beat yourself up when this happens. You might actually be better off eating the slice (or two) of cake than depriving yourself then later trying to find something to compensate for having restricted yourself.

I used to go to this locally owned little general store. The bakery section smelled just like my grandma's kitchen. Regardless of whether I was hungry or not, I'd buy a fresh cinnamon roll, just like the ones my grandma used to make. Instantly I was taken back. Eating and smelling the cinnamon roll brought comfort. I felt like a carefree child at Grandma's house again.

You might find yourself in a situation where you're a guest in the home of someone whose culture serves and feeds guests as a sign of love. Even if you ate just before you arrived, declining to eat wouldn't just be rude, it could be perceived as an insult or that you would be rejecting their affection.

Darlene was supposed to go to her neighbor Peyton's house early one Saturday afternoon and help her choose paint colors and fabric for her new drapes. She was dragging behind schedule that morning and ate a really late breakfast right before she left. When she arrived, she discovered she wasn't there to help choose colors and fabrics. Her friend was throwing her a surprise wedding shower with none other than a fully catered lunch from her favorite restaurant. She was the guest of honor! How could she not eat?

There are countless reasons why we might eat when we're not hungry. It's okay. All these scenarios are just things. It's what we think about these things that give them meaning. Choose to think something that helps you feel, do, and get what best serves you.

Just like I don't care for the term *thought loop*, I really don't like the term *emotional eating*. Wouldn't it be more accurate to say we really just want more control when we're experiencing unpleasant feelings and absentmindedly or carelessly overeat then feel guilty about it?

Sometimes we eat instead of feeling, and that is one of the reasons emotional eating has such a bad reputation. We turn to food to rescue us when we really need something else. Sometimes we eat because we're bored, and food becomes a source of delight. Darlene often used food as a form of pleasure at the tedious monthly committee meetings she was required to attend at her previous job. She hated just sitting as they went on and on, all day long, talking about nonsense and never reaching a decision. She needed some level of excitement, so she ate Danish pastries, candies, crackers, whatever was available.

Sometimes we use food for gratification when we don't like the task we're working on, or we've been working on it for too long. When Darlene was studying for her real estate exam, she'd buy big bags of M&M's and Skittles and allowed herself to eat them only if she was studying. If we're being completely honest, there were more than a few times while I was writing this book when I'd either sat too long or hit a block and found myself staring blankly at the screen, then I'd reach for some inspiration from Ben & Jerry.

When I was four years old, I fell and split my chin open on the basement floor. My mom rushed me to the emergency room where they stitched it closed. The day I had to go back and have the stitches removed, I remember my mom bought me a bag of Circus Peanuts, my favorite candy at the time. She opened the bag and set it on the front seat of the car between us and told me I could eat as many as I wanted. Mind you, back then bags of candy were much larger than they are today, and small children sat in the front seat of the car (without a seatbelt). I ate the entire bag. I remember how good they tasted and how excited I was. It was a big deal. I never got to eat as many as I wanted. What I don't remember, though, is experiencing any discomfort, physically or emotionally, from having the stitches removed from my chin. Those Circus Peanuts did a great job of distracting my thoughts in that scary situation.

When you do these kinds of things, acknowledge them and decide what meaning you want to attach to them. They are just actions that become facts. You choose how you're going to think and feel, so pick something that helps you feel, do, and get what best serves you.

HERE IS WHERE INTUITIVE EATING SHOWS UP TO COMBAT WHAT WE CONSIDER EMOTIONAL EATING

One of the biggest concerns I hear when someone starts Intuitive Eating is they can't trust themselves. If they're allowed to eat whatever they want, they're afraid they'll never stop. And they consider that endless eating a form of emotional eating. I don't agree. Give yourself full permission to eat as much as you want. If you love Skittles then put them near the TV, in your purse, in the car, on your desk, in the drawer, and near the bed. Put them everywhere. When you want one, have one. Before long, knowing you can have them whenever you want, you'll discover you really don't want them that often. I know, that's hard to believe. Check out this story and tell me if it sounds at all familiar.

Way before she became a realtor, Darlene had an amazing job with one of the most sought-after companies. They had harsh rules, and Darlene, along with every other employee in the company, made damn sure they followed them. One of those rules was absolutely no fraternizing between employees. It was strictly forbidden for employees to text, call, friend, follow, or see each other outside of work. Darlene didn't mind, well, until she met Stew. They made a quick connection, and before long, the chemistry was obvious. As the months went by, their connection became stronger and stronger. All Darlene wanted to do was be around Stew. She hated going home on Fridays, and she loved going back to work on Mondays. She just wanted to spend more time with him. All she thought about was Stew. She thought about Stew when she was cleaning the house. She thought about Stew when she watched TV. She even found herself rolling over in her sleep at night and dreaming about Stew being there beside her. There wasn't a doubt in her mind, she had totally fallen for Stew. Then one Monday morning, she eagerly showed up to work as she always did, and Stew wasn't there. He had resigned. Her heart sank until lunchtime when she ran into him at the deli across from her office. They were no longer restricted from seeing each other anytime they wanted. Needless to say, they hooked up. For the next several months, Darlene had a lot of Stew. She had Stew in the morning. She had Stew on her lunch break. She had Stew in the car. She had Stew on the couch in front of the TV. She had Stew on the floor. She had Stew in the middle of the night. She just wanted as much Stew as she could get. Fast forward eleven years, three active kids, Stew's hectic job, a cat, two small dogs to walk, dinner, dishes, and laundry, Darlene still loves Stew, and she still has Stew from time to time, she just doesn't have as much Stew as she did back when she was first allowed to have as much Stew as she wanted.

Anytime you give yourself unrestricted permission to have what you want, you're probably going to want a lot of it in the beginning. After a while, the excitement wears off. Not only that but food also activates the pleasure center of the brain much less when it's eaten more frequently. Again, this book isn't intended for anyone diagnosed with an addiction disorder or currently in an addiction treatment program.

HOW TO STOP USING FOOD TO FEED OUR FEELINGS

When you feel like you're using food for avoidance or to feed your feelings, ask yourself two questions:

- What am I feeling?
- What do I need?

When Darlene sat in those endless meetings, she was bored as hell. She felt like she was wasting her time, and she turned to food to get rid of the boredom. Except eating didn't satisfy her need. Whether it's food or any other tool, if it's not meeting your need, it's not going to work. The need will remain. Darlene needed to feel like she was accomplishing something during these meetings. Participation and food weren't meeting that need. She could plan to bring along a mindless activity. Some of Darlene's colleagues brought knitting projects, and their needles rapidly clinked away throughout the meeting. Darlene swore some of these women completed entire king-sized blankets in just a single meeting!

When I'd hit a writing block, what I really needed was a break and a change of scenery. My head was clogged, and my body was stiff. Sure, it was reassuring that Ben & Jerry were willing to help me out, but that wasn't what I needed. Moving around, taking a walk, even putting in a load of laundry hit the spot better than support from my two dear friends.

Having a list of things that you can pick from when you need a break is a lot easier than trying to come up with something to do when you're in the middle of needing it. The list could include things like taking a bath, a walk, a nap, or calling a friend.

Take a minute now and create a list of things you can do when you need a little break, and turning to food, while pleasant as that might taste, isn't exactly what you need to fix what's going on at that moment.

You may discover you actually do need a little quality time with Ben & Jerry and that's fine. If you're going to spend time with them, treat them as you would any other guest. Avoid distractions and give them your attention and enjoy the pleasure of their company.

FIGURE OUT WHAT'S REALLY GOING ON

Do you need to spend a few minutes experiencing whatever it is you're feeling? It's okay to have an unpleasant feeling and to notice it for a while. Sometimes that's all it takes for it to go away. Is Mean Girl slinging cruel comments, encouraging you to bury your feelings by eating? This is a time we really need to separate from Mean Girl. If you're not at a place where you can change or challenge her, then create a new voice. Use your imagination and say things to yourself that you would say to a friend. What would you say if your friend was experiencing whatever discomfort you are right now? Write it down and read it back to yourself as if she were saying it to you.

WHY IS SHE DOING THIS? WHY DOES MEAN GIRL TELL US TO EAT?

Mean Girl wants you to think you're not strong enough to handle your feelings. Remember how scary Jack Nicholson was in the movie *A Few Good Men* when he screamed, "You can't handle the truth"? That's what Mean Girl says, "You can't handle your feelings." Dealing with your feelings would enable you to grow and become a stronger person. That's unchartered territory for Mean Girl. She'd rather scare you into thinking you can't handle your feelings because she doesn't want to deal with discomfort. She's going to encourage you to mask it with the soothing taste of Lindt chocolate. Ask her, "What else can we do right now?" In the beginning, she may not have an answer. With practice, she'll have a new repertoire of ideas.

The more you know yourself, the more you can help yourself. I mentioned above speaking to yourself like you would to a friend. Get to know yourself, so you know how to talk to yourself. Also, getting to know yourself makes you a stronger person and more confident in your choices. The more confident you are, the easier it is to get out of your default cycles and release yourself from the power of Mean Girl.

Take some time, sit down, and get to know yourself. Ask questions about yourself:

- Where's your favorite vacation spot?
- What's your favorite movie?
- What's something unique about you most people don't know (that's not on your Facebook page)?

- What's the scariest thing you ever did?

As you answer those questions, go deeper and ask yourself:

- Why?
- Really?
- Is that true?

Recently, I answered a question in a Facebook group, "What's your favorite color?" Without hesitation, I answered "pink." Then a follow-up question came, "What do you have that's pink?" I started thinking about it. Almost nothing. There isn't anything in my house that's pink. Aside from a few pink shirts and some nail polish, and the fact that I lean toward cakes and cookies with pink frosting, very little pink. Most of my clothes are black, white, blue, or brown. I don't own a pink handbag or shoes (I did have white and pink sneakers but lost them in the fire). When I got married a few years ago, there wasn't any pink in my wedding. So why did I so quickly say pink is my favorite color? Because pink has always been my favorite color. When I was little, my room was decorated in pink, even the shag carpet. My clothes, my backpack, my hair clips were all pink. If pink was an option, that's what I chose. I'm not a little girl anymore, and I've grown out of pink. But the file in my brain for "favorite color" still has pink tucked inside. I still like it; it's a fun color, but no longer my favorite, and I wasn't even aware of that.

Take out a sheet of paper, or go to my website www. julieglynn.com, and download the Getting to Know Yourself Worksheets and answer the questions.

Once you've completed these exercises and gotten to know yourself a little better, go back and take some time to connect with Mean Girl. Show her you're strong enough to handle your feelings. Acknowledge her role in helping you develop into the person that you are. Then break out of the default cycle she's trying to trap you in that looks like this:

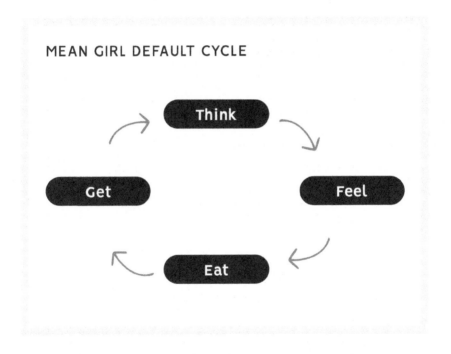

MEAN GIRL DEFAULT CYCLE

Here's an example:

One sunny Saturday afternoon, young Darlene sat home alone feeling sorry for herself because she didn't have a boyfriend to hang out with. Mean Girl pointed out that she should get used to being alone. She was lazy and pathetic. She didn't even try to go out and meet people. It was just as well; she had nothing to offer a relationship anyway. So, she sat on the couch and ate Whoopie Pies, candy, ice cream, chips, soda, popcorn, cookie dough, anything she could lay her hands on. One right after the other. She knew she'd feel physically ill from eating as much sugar, flour, and dairy as she did. She didn't care. She already felt like crap emotionally, so did it matter if she also felt like crap physically? Here was the Mean Girl Default Cycle:

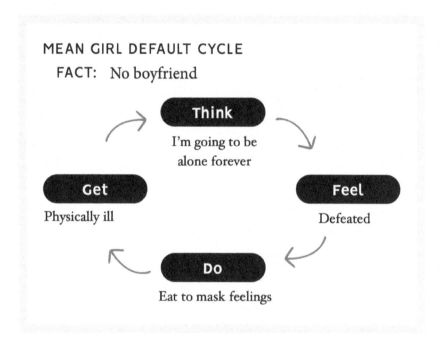

We want to stop that default cycle by creating a new Silver Lining Cycle. These are some examples of questions you could ask yourself:

"What do I want to DO?" (Answer: Experience my feelings and grow as a person.)

Follow up question: So, what do I want to do instead?

(Answer: I could look at the list I created in this chapter of ideas for when I need a break.)

Question: What will I do? Something new or something from the list? (Answer: I could take a walk, call a friend.)

Question: What do I need to FEEL in order to do that? (Answer: Self-compassion.)

Question: What do I need to THINK in order to feel that? (Answer: I need to think that I have plenty to add to any relationship.)

Follow-up question: How do you know you have plenty to add to a relationship? (Answer: Go look at my list of positive qualities I created in chapter 11.)

It's invaluable to have completed the planning-ahead activity mentioned above. Things are going to happen when we feel rejected, defeated, or lost. When Mean Girl comes knocking, trying to build up those negative feelings and drag you down, you can tap into those discoveries from the activities you've already done and use them to comfort and reassure both yourself and Mean Girl. It's not only empowering but it's also a form of self-compassion. The more you acknowledge and talk with Mean Girl, the more manageable she becomes. The more you increase your level of compassion for both Mean Girl and yourself, the more in touch you are with what you're feeling and what you need.

* * *

ACTIVITY:

When you feel like you're using food for avoidance or to feed your feelings, ask yourself two questions:

- What am I feeling?
- What do I need?

Having a list of things that you can pick from when you need a break is a lot easier than trying to come up with something to do when you're in the middle of needing it. The list could include things like taking a bath, a walk, a nap, or calling a friend.

Use your imagination and say things to yourself that you would say to a friend. What would you say if your friend was experiencing whatever discomfort you are right now? Write it down and read it back to yourself as if she were saying it to you.

Take a minute now and create a list of things you can do when you need a little break, and turning to food, while pleasant as that might taste, isn't exactly what you need to fix what's going on at that moment.

Take some time, sit down, and get to know yourself. Ask questions about yourself:

- Where's your favorite vacation spot?
- What's your favorite movie?

- What's something unique about you most people don't know (that's not on your Facebook page)?
- What's the scariest thing you ever did?

As you answer those questions, go deeper and ask yourself:

- Why?
- Really?
- Is that true?

MEAN GIRL STRATEGY:

When you get into a situation where Mean Girl encourages you to feed your feelings, and you really don't want anything to eat, ask her, "What else can we do right now?" She'll be startled by the question. The more you get to know yourself and do the activities above, the better she'll be able to come up with some new ideas.

❧ 13 ☙

MEAN GIRL LIE:

I'M ALWAYS GOING TO BE A FAILURE

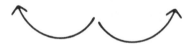

It's been a long journey for Darlene. She put in the work and changed her relationship with her body, her thoughts about food, and the way she sees herself in the world around her. She has journals full of lists and activities she completed like the ones mentioned in this book. Most importantly, she and Mean Girl have joined forces and become a team.

The first thing Darlene did was change Mean Girl's name. She thought long and hard for just the right name. She gave it as much consideration as she did when she named her children. She finally selected the name Honey. It's sweet yet can also create a huge sticky mess if not cared for and handled properly. As their relationship improved and they were more honest and supportive with one another, Honey told Darlene, in her own defense, "How could you ever expect me to be anything but a mean girl when that's how you referred to me?" Darlene knew Honey was right.

DARLENE NEEDS A NEW DRESS

Darlene doesn't miss the days she used to stand half-naked, nearly in tears, in front of the mirror surrounded by mounds of clothes she'd tried on, removed, and thrown to the floor. It was bad enough she hated her body, trying to find something to wear was like the story of Goldilocks. Nothing was ever just right. She didn't like the way it fit, the way it looked, or the way it made her feel.

For years, Darlene had a very ineffective method of choosing clothes when she went shopping. Her first criterion was price. Next, she considered how cute it was. After that, she checked the size, not the fit, but the size on the tag. She'd often purchase garments that rated high in those three categories. She rarely ever considered how well the clothes actually fit or how they looked on her. She figured they might eventually fit someday, right? As a result, her closet was filled with great-priced cute clothes that didn't really fit. No wonder she had so much trouble finding something to wear.

Once she started showing compassion and acceptance for the body she has today, she started dressing for her current size and wearing clothes that fit and felt good. That meant she had to change her shopping habits.

Now when Darlene goes shopping and finds something she likes, she grabs one in three different sizes. The size she thinks she is and then one a size up and one a size down. In the dressing room, she picks one, without looking at the size, turns her back to the mirror, and puts it on.

Without looking in the mirror, she will reach up high, reach to the front, reach side to side, reach down to her toes, do a few squats, take a little walk, lift her knees to her nose, wiggle around, and sit for a minute if there's a chair or a bench.

During all of this, she pays attention to how it feels:

Is it tight?
Is it loose?
Does it pinch?
Does it pull?
Does it dig?
Does it itch?
Does it stick?

If it's not completely comfortable, she doesn't even bother looking in the mirror. She takes it off and puts it in the discard pile. If it feels super comfortable on her body and passes the test, she turns around and looks in the mirror. After she considers how it looks and how she feels wearing it, she decides whether or not to add it to her wardrobe. That's exactly how Darlene selected the dress she wore to her high school reunion.

DARLENE FINALLY ATTENDS A HIGH SCHOOL REUNION

Darlene was so glad she decided to go to her class reunion. She felt amazing in her new dress as she danced with her friends. She took a break and wandered over to the bar for a drink. As she was waiting for the bartender, she heard a voice behind her say, "Well, if it isn't Darlene, the prettiest girl I ever knew."

Had she had a drink in her hand, she probably would've dropped it when she spun around and saw Clyde right there on the stool next to her. How did he even recognize her? She thought she was fat last time he saw her. She sure didn't look the same now, and how many years did she wish she was that size again?

He went on to tell her he'd attended every class reunion since graduation hoping he'd run into her.

"Oh?" she asked. "What happened with you and Bonita? I heard you got married right after high school?"

Apparently, that didn't last very long. Bonita left shortly after their wedding when she discovered Clyde didn't want children.

Again, had she had a drink in her hand, she probably would've dropped it. Clyde didn't want children? That was interesting; she never knew that. But then how would she considering Bonita didn't even find out until after their wedding. That information might have saved buckets of tears and the heartache she suffered back in the day. Darlene had three children. If she was going to make a list of ten reasons their breakup was a gift, she could easily put her children's names on lines one, two, and three.

Poor Clyde. Here he was, middle-aged, single, with no children. From what she gathered, he may have been sitting all alone on that barstool much more frequently than just the previous reunions she hadn't attended.

It was difficult trying to have a conversation with Clyde. He had very little to say about his life, interests, or career. Instead, he was stuck in the past and just wanted to relive old memories talking about things Darlene had long forgotten and didn't want to relive.

She quickly started looking for an opportunity to escape. Clyde didn't want any part of that and kept trying to touch her, suggesting they find someplace where they could be alone together. What a disappointment. He obviously didn't care that she was married. (There was a quick number four on her list.) She found an opening and ducked away when a large crowd gathered nearby. She shook her head as she left. What she just saw certainly didn't match the image she mourned for way back when her future with Clyde abruptly ended.

Honey piped up with regret and said, "I can't believe we cried a single tear over him." Then she turned jovial and said, "But did you hear him say you were pretty? Score one for Darlene!" Darlene chuckled in agreement, even as she felt bad for Clyde, all alone and so desperate, he's trying to hook up with a married woman.

Darlene gathered her stuff, hugged, and said goodbye to her friends then gave the DJ a big tip. As she headed to leave, she thought this was clearly a situation where things turned out exactly the way they were supposed to. As she opened the door to leave, the song she requested came on, and she heard Garth Brooks sing, "Sometimes I thank God for unanswered prayers..."

As Darlene walked to her car, she said aloud, "Honey, when I get home, I'm going to add you to my list of things to be grateful for. I couldn't have done this tonight without you."

DARLENE AND STEW

It took a lot of baby steps and a long time before Darlene finally got her first real estate client that subsequently resulted in the sale of a property. As a pilot, Stew traveled a lot but was scheduled to arrive back home the same day as the closing of her first sale. They planned to celebrate that night at her favorite restaurant. She was looking forward to eating her favorite foods from its menu and enjoying a celebratory piece of its famous coconut cake.

Right after they ordered, Darlene was taken aback when Stew suggested she stop dabbling in real estate. He went on to point out she'd been a stay at home mom with the kids for over nine years, and he felt it was time for her to get a regular job that provided a regular income.

She didn't understand. They didn't need the money, and she didn't have any other job skills or much education besides the year's worth of college courses she took right after high school. She asked him for an explanation. He told her he'd been fired. Fired? That didn't make sense. She asked, "Why were you fired?"

"I was fired because I had an affair," he responded.

It couldn't be true. This must be some kind of a joke. He's a pilot, why would he get fired for having an affair?

Stew went on to explain that it was a little worse than it sounded. He didn't just have a secret rendezvous. Other pilots and employees from the airline reported witnessing inappropriate sexual behavior he had in a hotel hot tub with more than one female member of the flight crew. He started to describe other indiscretions in airports and on the planes, but Darlene stopped him. She didn't want to hear anymore.

All sorts of thoughts were bouncing around in her head, but mostly, "This can't be happening." "What am I going to do?" "I'm never going to find a silver lining in this mess." Maybe just hearing the words *silver lining* brought to her attention the fact that the commission check tucked away in her handbag was made out in her name. She decided as soon as she dropped the kids off at school the next day, she'd open her own account at a new bank and deposit her check.

She couldn't deny her feelings of disbelief, anger, betrayal, sadness, fear, and uncertainty. It was going to take a lot of strength to get through this. Then she found another silver lining. Thank goodness this didn't happen a few years ago when she was at war with herself. It was going to be rough for

Darlene. She forced herself to hold it together as best as she could for the sake of her children.

The first thing she did was kick Stew out of the house. She then spent the next several weeks dragging herself out of bed just long enough to put on a happy face and get the kids off to school. Then she'd hurry home and either go back to bed and cry until the bus dropped the kids off, or she'd make pancakes or homemade cookies and enjoy the pleasure of the sweet taste in her mouth.

Occasionally she'd find some moments where she felt ready to start moving forward. When that happened, the first thing she did was sit down and write a letter to her sister Mellie, as she learned in chapter 12. She wrote down all the things she would tell Mellie if her husband, Jack, had betrayed her and destroyed her family and future the way Stew had done to Darlene. She loved Mellie so much, it was easy writing that letter explaining how Mellie didn't deserve what she was going through. She released a lot of pent-up anger in her letter, including how horrible she thought Jack was for what he did. Of course, she read and reread the letter back to herself many times over the next several months.

She grabbed her journal with the ongoing list of positive things in her life that she had started in chapter 4.

A few years back, she created a new morning routine based on what she'd worked on in chapter 6. She kept adding to her positive list on a daily basis, including things she had to be grateful for. As she read through the list, she realized she wasn't in the space right now to come up with any new things to add to the list, so she was glad she had created the list previously. As she read through the items on list now, she nodded her head in agreement. She still had things to be grateful for in spite of the heartache she was experiencing.

As she gathered the resources she'd created to help herself, she realized it never crossed her mind that the size of her ass had anything to do with her current situation. In fact, she felt pretty confident that she never did anything to deserve this, and Stew clearly was not the man she thought he was.

Of course, in the beginning, Honey thought it was best if they just stayed in bed for like the next twenty-five years. When Darlene seriously questioned, "What are we going to do?" Honey was quick to respond, "Stew needs to suffer." Darlene agreed, but she wasn't one to intentionally cause another person pain. Even though she felt like it was Stew's fault, she wasn't going to let his actions ruin her life. She was going to continue the personal growth journey she had already started. She decided right then and there she was going to stand on her own two feet and support her three kids. She would never rely on Stew, or any other man for that matter, ever again.

But what was she going to do? She hadn't worked in nearly ten years. Selling real estate was much too unpredictable for her current situation. She needed a career. Where could she add value in the world. She looked in her journal and found the list she created from chapter 6. She noticed some similarities on the list. She gave it careful consideration and thought for a while. She was inspired by her sister Louisa who loved her job as a nurse. Plus, she enjoyed the science classes she took the year she was in college, so she did some research and enrolled in nursing school.

DARLENE GOES BACK TO SCHOOL

Darlene knew this was going to be hard, not just academically, but she knew what it was like when Honey wanted her to stay home and keep from growing. She was determined. She pulled out the same strength she had dedicated to the years and years she spent dieting and exercising. The strength and determination she never even knew she had and probably wouldn't have been able to tap in to just a few short years ago.

She started working part-time at an extended care facility during the day and attending nursing school at night.

This was a very difficult time for Darlene. She was working her ass off and hurting at the same time. She was trying to juggle her own schoolwork while also trying to be the best mom she could be—attending dance recitals, PTA meetings, sporting events, hosting birthday parties.

She and Honey had a lot of conversations and played a lot of silly games during this trying time. It was hard every semester when Darlene walked into a new classroom for the first time. She had to fight feelings of intimidation and inferiority. She had to remind herself she had tested well on the entrance exam, and she received good grades on her assignments. She worked hard using the same small baby steps she used when she got her first real estate client.

She still spent a lot of nights lying awake fighting off thoughts that created worry and uncertainty. Every now and then she'd think, "I can't do this." But then she'd hear Honey say, "But you are doing it."

And so she did.

She graduated magna cum laude. She had so many things to be grateful for. She pulled it together in one of her darkest moments. She had unconditional support from the people in her life who care about her—her mom, her sisters Millie and Louise, and her friend Peyton. Her children continued to thrive with minimal disruption from the divorce. And she got an amazing nursing job at the local hospital.

JUST WHEN DARLENE THOUGHT EVERYTHING WAS PERFECT

A few years later, Darlene woke up a little lonely one bright sunny summer morning. It was quiet, and all three of her kids were away at camp for the week. She was lazy and moving around pretty slowly when she heard the beeping of a loud truck backing up.

She didn't give it much attention until she noticed a fully dressed man inside the fenced pool area of her small condo community and a tanker truck in the yard behind her unit that said Baxter Water on the side.

Nobody else was around, so she quickly threw on a pair of shorts and a t-shirt and went to investigate. Turns out, Baxter was there to fill the pool that had recently been drained and repaired. Darlene was so excited. Nobody was more eager than she to have the pool operational and ready to use again.

She spoke briefly with Baxter about the logistics and checked to see if he needed anything. Typically, she would have wandered off at that point, but instead of ending the conversation, it seemed natural to keep chatting while Baxter unraveled the hose from the truck and placed it into the pool.

At that point, Baxter just had to wait for the water to empty from the truck into the pool. Having nothing else to do and with the conversation still moving along, she pulled up a chair and sat with Baxter for a while.

The conversation flowed as smoothly as the water from the hose. Before she knew it, nearly an hour had passed, and the hose was sputtering air. As Baxter started reeling the hose back onto the truck, he explained that he would return after he refilled the truck.

He kind of stammered when he asked if she'd be there when he got back, indicating he would be leaving a box of pool supplies and didn't want anything to happen to them. Darlene was pretty sure that was a bogus excuse, and he just wanted to confirm he'd see her later. She hid her excitement and assured him she would be available when he returned.

She went to use the bathroom when she went back inside and nearly screamed in horror when she looked at herself in the mirror. She had thrown clothes on so quickly and gone outside, she hadn't done a thing with her hair. She hadn't so much as run a brush through it since she got up. She didn't have a bit of makeup on. Upon further inspection, her toes revealed she was way overdue for a pedicure, and the forest growing on her legs should have been addressed days ago.

She said, "I look a wreck."

Honey agreed, but assured, "Honestly, I don't think he noticed; if he did, he certainly didn't care."

Wow. She and Baxter just spent the past couple of hours chatting and flirting back and forth like high schoolers, and she was completely uninhibited by what she looked like. And it didn't appear that he cared.

What was she going to do now? She certainly couldn't take a shower and gussy herself up. That would be awkward. She decided to take a shower and put on clean clothes, which she was going to do anyway. Typically, she also would have freshened up her face and done something with her hair. She decided against it. She put on a pair of sneakers to cover her toes.

Because she didn't want to appear as excited and eager as she was, when Baxter was back, she waited nearly fifteen minutes before she moseyed out into the backyard. Soon another conversation struck up, and she was back sitting in the same chair she was in earlier. They laughed and talked until it looked like the pool might overflow.

As Baxter started reeling the hose back onto the truck, Darlene got up to leave. Before she wandered too far, he stopped her and asked if he could see her again. Of course she wanted to see him again. She accepted every invitation to spend time with him all the way up until he asked if she wanted to spend the rest of her life with him. She accepted that too.

Years later, they still laugh and giggle whenever someone asks how they first met. Baxter loves to tell the story, "I was doing my job one sunny morning when I saw this woman marching toward me in what looked like yesterday's clothes she picked up from the floor. Something about the way she held herself and the confidence that flowed from her, I could see, as plain as day, the beauty in her soul."

Darlene didn't think it was possible she could ever feel more loved, accepted, and beautiful. Then Baxter came along.

WANT MORE?

JOIN THE FACEBOOK GROUP

Become part of the community and connect with other readers of "if my ASS were smaller life would be perfect & other LIES Mean Girl in your head tells you" at www. facebook.com/groups/ifmyASSweresmaller. This is a sacred encouraging space for women to talk about how this book impacted their lives, share ideas and experiences, and support one another in their journey.

ENROLL IN THE ONLINE COURSE

Want a deeper dive into the activities in this book? More individualized attention? The opportunity to ask questions and collaborate with others?

Check out the the online Anti-diet, Intuitive Eating, Mean Girl Transformation Academy

This interactive membership community is filled with videos and activities to help you go deep and really transform your Mean Girl while embarking on your anti-diet, Intuitive Eating journey. Check it out at www.JulieGlynn.com

NEED SOMETHING MORE PERSONALIZED?

To learn more about incorporating the concepts of this book into your life through one-on-one coaching, to book me for your next event, podcast, seminar or if you have any other questions, I can be reached at:

JulieGlynn@yahoo.com

or

P.O. Box 63

Hanover, NH 03755

JOIN ME IN CREATING SOCIAL CHANGE

There were times when I walked into a room, scanned the crowd then realized I was the largest person in the group. How quickly my Mean Girl made me feel small and unworthy on the inside.

I wondered if anyone else ever had that experience, and if they did, was there something I could do to alleviate their discomfort? I came up with an idea. Wouldn't it be great if there was some kind of symbol or message to indicate love and acceptance of all people regardless of their appearance?

So I created one.

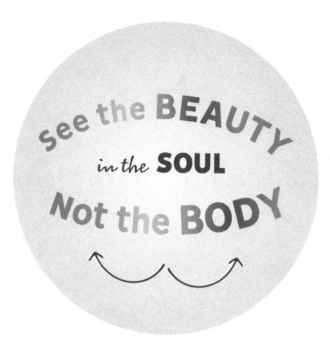

Wouldn't it be great to live in a world where everyone dives deeper than just the surface when they look at another person. A world where judgment based on size, shape or appearance doesn't exist. It is my hope you will join me in my effort to create social change by spreading the word and displaying this message. Let's remind everyone that beauty radiates outward from the soul, it doesn't rest on the surface. Visit my website, www.julieglynn.com and check out all the different ways you can display this message.

ACKNOWLEDGEMENTS

Initially I didn't want to include an acknowledgment page. How can I possibly acknowledge every one who played a part in the creation of this book? Because, let's face it, every single person I've come in contact with, every interaction I've encountered, whether good or bad, has impacted my life and shaped me into the person I am today. I didn't know where to draw the line. With that being said, I want to acknowledge all of you who've ever been part of my life. Thank you.

And to these people specifically:

Several years ago I attended a pretty extensive six month training. It involved 3 trips, airfare, hotels, and meals. It was expense, but it was worth it. I knew it was going to change my life. And that it did. I met my friend, Diane Riis. Diane is an author's coach and owner of Earth and Soul Coaching and Publishing, Inc. which helps authors create transformational books through coaching, editing, book design and marketing.

I don't know how she put up with me through this process, but I'm glad she did. Without her skills and expertise and unending patience, this book never would have happened.

Diane put me in touch with Andrea Schmidt, a-schmidt.com. Not only did Andrea design my cover, format the text, and create my graphics, she was instrumental in helping me with promotion and marketing. Most importantly she kept me calm and answered all my questions. I'm so grateful to have found her.

Like we haven't already spoke enough about how what we think determines how we feel, what we do and what we get I just have to include one more example. I've seen posts on Facebook like "I really don't know why I come here anymore, it's so angry and toxic." I seriously couldn't have written this book if it wasn't for Facebook. No, my acknowledgment isn't to Facebook. It's for all the amazing people I've met on Facebook because I refuse to get sucked into the toxicity. Whitney Sweet, Cindy Shames, Ashlee Renee, Soetkin De Boever, Beverly Riggs Garden, Vie Portland, Megan Bennett, Karen Daas, Morgan Faie, Joy Stephanos, Beth Allen, Nikki Williams Elswick, Elana Halpin Sardella, and Mariana Moll. I can 't thank all of you enough for your support, encouragement and feedback.

NOTES

NOTES

NOTES

NOTES

NOTES

NOTES

NOTES

NOTES